Jandi Beck

MISS I

MISS DIAGNOSED

◆

Unraveling Chronic Stress

Erin M. Bell with Foreword by Dr. Shawn Talbott, author of The Cortisol Connection

iUniverse, Inc.
New York Lincoln Shanghai

MISS DIAGNOSED
Unraveling Chronic Stress

Copyright © 2005 by Erin M. Bell

All rights reserved. No part of this book may be used or reproduced by any means, graphic, electronic, or mechanical, including photocopying, recording, taping or by any information storage retrieval system without the written permission of the publisher except in the case of brief quotations embodied in critical articles and reviews.

iUniverse books may be ordered through booksellers or by contacting:

iUniverse
2021 Pine Lake Road, Suite 100
Lincoln, NE 68512
www.iuniverse.com
1-800-Authors (1-800-288-4677)

The information contained in this book is for educational purposes only. It is a personal account of the author's own medical experiences. It should not be used as a means of diagnosis or treatment of any illness. Consult a qualified medical professional for individual health concerns.

ISBN-13: 978-0-595-35688-1 (pbk)
ISBN-13: 978-0-595-80165-7 (ebk)
ISBN-10: 0-595-35688-5 (pbk)
ISBN-10: 0-595-80165-X (ebk)

Printed in the United States of America

To my siblings:
Tammy, Dan, Katie, and Gloria
—this is for you!

It is highly dishonorable for a reasonable soul to live in so divinely built a mansion as the body she resides in, altogether unacquainted with the exquisite structure of it.
—Robert Boyle, 1627–1691

Contents

Foreword... xv
Introduction xvii

Chapter 1 A Foundation of Stress 1
Chapter 2 Denied!....................................... 4
Chapter 3 The Incurable Woman 10
- *Diagnosis: Overuse of Painkillers*....................... *10*
- *Diagnosis: Hypoglycemia* *12*
- *Diagnosis: Candida Syndrome* *13*
- *Diagnosis: Sleep Disorder—Insomnia* *15*
- *Diagnosis: Tension Headaches*............................ *18*
- *Diagnosis: Tinnitus*..................................... *21*

Chapter 4 Chronic Stress—Depression's Evil Twin! 25
- *Seek and Ye Shall Find*.................................. *27*
- *Still at War*.. *29*
- *Understanding Stress* *33*
- *Cortisol: The Mystery Hormone* *35*
- *So…What Is Cortisol?* *38*
- *Who Knew?*... *42*

Chapter 5 Going to the Root of the Problem.............. 45
- *Dissecting Stress and Distress*.......................... *45*
- *Do Kids Have Stress?*.................................... *51*
- *Masking the Problem* *52*
- *Chronic Stress vs. Depression*........................... *53*

- *Did Cortisol Make Me Do It?* *55*
- *Feeding Stress!.* *57*
- *The Immune System* *61*
- *Cortisol and Sleep* *62*

Chapter 6 Controversial Candida 64
- *Cortisol and Candida* *67*
- *"You Have to Seek It Out"* *68*
- *Could Candida Be Your Problem?.* *69*
- *Candida and Chronic Fatigue Syndrome* *71*

Chapter 7 What Is Stressing Us? 72
- *Prisoners of Time* *72*
- *"Just Take a Pill!".* *74*
- *We Lose Control.* *75*
- *Sisters of Perpetual Motion* *77*
- *You've Come a Long Way Baby—(but…Just Keep Going)!* ... *78*
- *Toxic People!* *80*
- *Who Are "The Joneses" Anyway?* *81*
- *The Pressure.* *83*
- *Present: Tense!* *84*
- *We're Overworked* *86*
- *(Body) Image is Everything!.* *91*

Chapter 8 Simplify 94

Chapter 9 The Wisdom of Self-Education and Prevention 96
- *An Ounce of Prevention…* *98*
- *A New Attitude!* *100*
- *Natural Approach to a Natural Phenomenon* *101*
- *Natural Medicine.* *102*
- *Total Health* *105*
- *Try Sailing!* *106*

Chapter 10 Conclusion.. 109

REFERENCES..113
APPENDIX   Suggested Readings..........................127

Acknowledgments

I would like to thank the many people who helped me make this book a reality:

- My God and Lord, "The Great Physician," for giving me the key to unlock the mystery toward my good health.

- My husband, Ben—thank you for all your love and support.

- Dr. Shawn Talbott, for your contribution in the foreword address, as well as for providing private commentary. I will forever appreciate the encouragement, support, and enthusiasm you provided throughout my writing this book.

- Samuel Thomas, "The Word Whisperer," for your editorial assistance. Thank you for helping me form glittering gems from lumps of coal!

- My sister, Tammy, "The Midwife," for your inspiration, your editorial advice, and your tireless, listening ear.

- My beloved "fur-babies" (my cats), for your unconditional affection during the long hours spent at my computer while writing this book.

- The women who participated in my study group—including my wonderful friends at FirefightersWives.com—you girls are the best!

- Dr. Uwaya Erdmann, ND, for your editorial advice and support.

- Dr. Michael Biamonte, for private commentary.

- Dr. Richard Earle, for private commentary.
- Kristin and the staff at iUniverse.

Foreword

It is with great pleasure that I write this foreword for Erin Bell's outstanding personal account of her own health odyssey in *Miss Diagnosed*. As a lifestyle researcher, speaker, and author, I have spent the last decade educating health professionals and the public about the damaging health effects of chronic stress. Although my teachings are able to reach audiences on an intellectual level (so they understand the hows and whys of stress being "bad" for them), Ms. Bell has crafted here an extraordinary emotional account of her own personal travails with chronic stress and the ravages that such a battle may bring.

I am certain that readers will find, as I did, a bit of themselves described in Ms. Bell's search for a proper diagnosis of her health condition. Misdiagnosis after misdiagnosis leads Ms. Bell to discover on her own what many health professionals are only now beginning to appreciate—that chronic stress and cortisol exposure have wide-ranging health effects across all systems of the body.

In many ways, chronic stress and cortisol exposure can be implicated in the cause and course of almost every "modern" disease that we know of today, from heart disease, to cancer, to osteoporosis, to obesity, and diabetes. Cortisol, the body's primary stress hormone, is often referred to by stress physiologists as the "Death Hormone" because of its close association with tissue breakdown, metabolic dysfunction, and the very aging process itself.

Erin Bell's story in *Miss Diagnosed* exposes some of the scientific/medical basis of chronic stress and disease, but even more importantly, it brings a very personal angle to the daily situations experienced by millions of men and women. These people ask themselves why they're so tired and depressed, have no sex drive, are gaining weight, and can't remember where they left their keys—along with a dozen other annoying symptoms that can get dismissed or chalked up to being "in your head" by some medical professionals. Ms. Bell's story helps us recognize that these are all symptoms of chronic stress—and even better, she uses herself as an example of how we can live and thrive in our stressful, modern world.

Shawn M. Talbott, PhD, FACSM

Author, *The Cortisol Connection—Why Stress Makes You Fat & Ruins Your Health* (Hunter House, 2002); *The Cortisol Connection Diet—The Breakthrough Program to Control Stress and Lose Weight* (Hunter House, 2004)

Salt Lake City, UT

June 2005

Introduction

Miss Diagnosed is not a book about a misdiagnosis of a particular illness. It is a book about me being diagnosed with many different symptoms of a problem that I came to understand on my own. I wrote this book because when I was looking for answers to my health questions, I could not find something that would guide me where I needed to go—to the root of my problems. This is not just another book about stress and stress management. I wrote this book to help others understand the phenomenon of chronic stress and its effects on your body and to encourage readers to educate themselves about their health. Dr. David Posen writes in *The Little Book of Stress Relief*, "Stress can manifest itself in a dozen ways...most people have five or ten symptoms characteristic for *them*...if we learn to recognize our individual stress profile, [we can become better at detecting it]." "Identifying stress is the first step to doing something about it."[1] What you choose to do about the stress in your life is your decision. We all experience stress, but do we know what it's *really* doing to us?

I am not a doctor, and I do not have any expertise on the subject of stress. I have no professional medical training. I have not written from a medical point of view, but rather a personal point of view—the point of view that most of us can all relate to.

Taber's Cyclopedic Medical Dictionary defines stress "a narrowing"[2] and *The Random House Dictionary* defines it as "physical, mental, or emotional tension."[3]

Neither definition sounds very comforting. The narrowing definition presents the picture of being confined. It reminds me of a particular situation in which my own stress levels climb: being on a multi-lane highway with fast-moving traffic when suddenly all the traffic has to merge into one lane. This can be very frustrating. Miles and miles of agitated drivers crammed into one lane moving at a snail's pace. Have you ever been in this situation? Have you ever noticed the reactions of the drivers around you? Fists slam on dashboards, ties and buttons loosen, sweat glands activate, and angry murmurs form on lips. Cell phones promptly pop out everywhere as disappointed commuters make hasty calls to explain the delay. Everyone is frustrated, impatient, and worried about being late. I know I get just as irritated as the next person does when this happens to me. This is one scenario in which you can actually *see* stress at work—affecting the people around you. But, what about the stress we cannot see?

We live in a fast-paced world full of wide-widths, broad-spectrums, generous proportions, and "biggie-sizes." Narrowing just doesn't cut it! My interpretation of stress is that it limits our abilities and our health—forcing us to squeeze into circumstances in our physical, mental, or emotional lives that make us uncomfortable. Stress is not just a state of mind; it is something that sets up camp in your body! It can affect all areas of your life—especially your health. It is also a broad and loose term that affects each individual differently. Stress itself is not an illness, but rather, a precursor to many illnesses and conditions. We often treat the symptoms but neglect the root of the problem.

Stress is a main contributor to women's health issues. Stress contributes to diseases like arthritis, breast cancer, immune system disorders, osteoporosis, heart disease, depression, and "mystery" illnesses like fibromyalgia and chronic fatigue syndrome.[4] Stress was also a primary contributor to the many symptoms I suffered; however, I never thought of stress as being a basis for disease. Like most everyone, I thought stress was something you just had to deal with. However, I did not learn this overnight. Looking back, I recognize the process of myriad symptoms that had me wandering nomadically to doctors for years looking for answers to my problems. Diagnosis after diagnosis, I was still searching for answers more than a decade later. Chronic stress was killing me, perhaps slowly, but eventually it would have made a statistic out of me. The statistics are nothing short of frightening—especially for women.

I wrote this book to appeal to women more than to men, but men could very well gain knowledge about how to control the effects of chronic stress in their lives as well. Since we all experience stress to some degree, we don't think of it as having the capacity to deteriorate our lives like cancer might or disrupt our ability to enjoy our lives, like diabetes, for instance. We really do not understand how stress actually affects us and what it actually does to our bodies. Like the thinning ozone layer or increasing taxes, we just live with it. Women, in particular, are living high-stress lifestyles without completely understanding how it is affecting them. They are often aware of how they feel under stress, but do not realize how it could be ruining their health.

My story is not about what I know; it's about how I found out what I *didn't* know.

It is my intention to share my knowledge and understanding about my own health problems so that it may inspire others to help themselves. If you are reading this book and find yourself saying, "That's me, I feel just like that," or if you've been told your problems are psychosomatic or "all in your head," then read on to understand why you might be feeling this way. You might just discover that you have been sharing center stage with me—*Miss Diagnosed*.

1

A Foundation of Stress

Stress can begin early in life for some, but we generally do not think of stress as being a child's problem. When children feel stress, we assume they can talk to their teddy bear or draw a picture to get over it. As teenagers, we often tell each other to "get over it" as we try to release pent up stress amongst our friends; moreover, the friendships we hold as teenagers determine to a great extent how we will deal with stress as adults; peer-pressured teen years are often some of the most stressful, which can cause lifelong scars and damage. These years often lay the cornerstones of our future, both the good and the bad. For teenagers, stress could likely be defined as a bad hair day or a lunch-hour breakup with a prom date. At least, that was how it seemed when I was in high school in the mid 1980s. Most of my peers probably did not start to experience increased or chronic stress until adulthood. Yet, for me, life unraveled somewhat differently.

I felt different, even estranged sometimes, although I would never reveal this to my friends and peers. I was sixteen when I left home. Home was not an environment I felt I could stay in throughout my teenage years. My childhood was marked with fear and uncertainty. Punishment—that was often physical and termed as "discipline"—rigid Catholic doctrines, poverty, gambling, and alcoholism prevailed. Anger and resentment lingered from our mother's own childhood. We lived a nomadic lifestyle. It seemed as though we could never really find "our home." It was like constantly living on high alert. Consequently, my siblings and I found strength among one another and looked out for one another. We evaded apprehension and social disgrace among our extended family by keeping silent about our troubled days.

Childhood was very unpredictable. Although our family celebrated special occasions and holidays lavishly with a strong sense of family connectedness, everyday life was marked with repeated episodes of turmoil and insecurity.

It may have seemed somewhat unconventional back then for me to be leaving so young, but it felt like my only choice. Four days after my sixteenth birthday, I left and moved in with my nineteen-year-old sister, who lived in a small town outside the city. When she was sixteen, pregnancy and marriage provided her an escape from our family's home life. As the eldest, she was the parentified sister. Basically, we were children raising children. I helped her raise her two little girls in their early years. My parents were outraged at my move, but I was legally old enough to leave without parental consent. I know now that, if I had not left when I did, this book would be filled with blank pages.

With the beginning of a new chapter in my life—freed from old restraints—new possibilities emerged. I was in a new town and a new school, and I could be anyone I wanted. Throughout high school, I may have appeared to the other kids as just another girl walking through the halls. I hid behind a mask of normalcy as I assume many troubled kids do, pretending that nothing was ever wrong at home. In reality, I had become my own parent at sixteen! This would seem like a dream come true to most teenagers; however, it's not all the fun and freedom it's cracked up to be. When you have to take care of yourself, even though you are still a kid, you soon learn to become an adult, rather quickly and prematurely. Unless you want to end up homeless, expelled from school, or sitting on a street corner, you've got to make up your mind to parent yourself as any responsible parent would.

I had to set limits for what I could do, or I would end up dislocated, perhaps even homeless. I also had to work extra hard because if I needed anything, I had to get it myself. When the other kids went home after school for their usual teenage rituals, I left the classroom for one of three part-time jobs. They were growing up as "normal" teenagers, and I was growing up an adult before my time.

I experienced the usual high school rituals of boyfriends and break-ups, proms and parties, and even some ribbing by other students who were not so comfortable with the idea of me being "the new girl." Most of them had grown up together and forged their friendships since elementary school. In this typical small town, there were preestablished cliques that were hard to break into. Here I was, merging into their territory. I did not have the security of childhood to find shelter in, and I struggled with this silently. Although I eventually found my niche, I felt alienated because I did not feel my friends in the teenaged world could understand that I was my own authority. I was with them, but in terms of my responsibilities, I wasn't one of them.

By the time I was nearly finished with high school, I was practically running on empty, but I completely ignored it. My school year was spent doing the best I could in class and working several part-time jobs on the side. My summers consisted of sixty-plus hour workweeks, serving as a waitress in local resorts—sometimes twelve and sixteen hours a day, as well as working in a nursing home and as a clerk in the town hall office. Still, I took my age for granted, had plenty of adrenaline to keep me going, and knew intuitively that if I did not do it all for myself, no one else would. Nonetheless, trying to go to school, juggling several jobs at once, and taking care of myself was taking its toll.

2

Denied!

I was excited about college because I actually got to slow down a little. I kept one part-time job and decided to focus more on my academics. Going into my courses, I felt positive that I would have more time to do better than I had done in high school. However, college ended up being even more of a disappointment than high school—not because I did not study hard, do my work, or apply myself, but seemingly, because of who I was. Let me explain. During my first semester of college, everything was new, and I took the time to get to know my instructors. The pace and workload were quite a contrast to high school. In class, some teachers were hard to follow, jumping from one tangent to the next. One instructor made my college life particularly stressful. The first time I went to her office to pick up an assignment, she mentioned that she knew who I was because my father had worked with her husband. I responded with a smile and a polite, "Oh, that's nice," and never gave it another thought. Not until I started to see my grades.

Throughout the next three semesters, I found myself continually arguing with this instructor because I felt she was marking me unfairly. I was at or above class average in all my courses except this particular one. My grades in her class were considerably lower than my other classes. It even prompted me to call my Dad to ask him about his working relationship with my instructor's husband. He explained that because they were in competitive sales, they had often locked horns with each other. Yet, to his knowledge, it was never personal. I did not think for a second that this teacher would use that against me. I was a college kid in her class—not a threat to her or her husband! To this day, I do not know if that was her problem with me, but she made my college life miserable.

It all came to a head during my last semester, when my marks were good again and at par with the rest of the class—except for one. One half-credit course stuck out on my final transcript like a sore thumb! I was shocked when I learned that the instructor that I had difficulty with all along had failed me. She would argue that I failed her, but I was a few percentage points shy of a pass in her class. Moreover, the final class average was disgracefully low at only 57 percent—a D! My other instructors stood wide-eyed with their jaws dropped. My interim reports from my other instructors boasted of a student who had "really shown interest" and was "making good progress"—one instructor even called me "gifted" and encouraged me to pursue more studies in my field. I appealed my marks with the instructor who had failed me, and I pleaded my case with her. It was my senior year; I was supposed to be on a podium accepting my diploma with hundreds of other students in a matter of weeks! She responded that I was not a dedicated student and failed to meet her requirements for a pass.

I took my dilemma to the college dean to seek justice for my situation and explained the difficulty I had had with this instructor. He was somewhat sympathetic. I showed him my transcript of my final marks, and he looked it over carefully. When he noticed the mark from my apparently failed course, he asked me, "What happened here, did you fall asleep in this class?" I explained that I thought the teacher "had it in for me" and that my other marks were too strong for me to have failed that miserably in just one course. He agreed that it seemed very unusual and highly suspicious that I would have earned such a low mark in just one course. He was also concerned that the class average was so low; however, he began to explain that he didn't want to open a can of worms with the instructor because she was up for a promotion, and it would look bad on her teaching record. I began to cry! I was shocked by his response! I would have preferred to meet the dean of the college while shaking his hand on graduation day. Here I was in tears in his office. I sobbed that I did not deserve this and did not care about the advancement of her career as much as I cared about owing thousands of dollars in student loans and leaving the college with no diploma! He shook his head apologetically and said there was nothing more he was willing to do. The college denied me my diploma. I would not graduate. My only choice of making up the missing half credit was to return in two years time when the same course would be offered again. I was devastated and in debt! I left his office and the college. On graduation day, I knew my classmates were wondering where I was. I thought I was a failure. That is what I believed. I was furious that the dean chose his staff over his student. For the next ten years, I believed I was a failure, hiding it from everyone that I did not get my college diploma. I slammed the academic door and resolved to never look back. All I could think about was that I was finished with college and had to find a job—diploma or not. I began to search for any job that did not require me to reveal my academic disgrace.

Shortly after college, the failure of my sister's teen marriage took her and her two children to another part of the province, leaving me to find my own place to live. I gathered up a black-and-white TV, a bed, a plastic lawn chair, and one saucepan to begin my life alone. I found my first apartment below a nice family. They were kind and even let me share their backyard swimming pool. I think they were a little concerned about me because I was only twenty years old. At one point, my landlord came down to my recently rented basement apartment, bringing some steaks and a bottle of hard whiskey. I guess I looked like I needed a stiff drink! He whipped up a BBQ on the patio, sat down, and asked me pointblank, "Erin, do you have any parents?" I told him yes and explained some of my reasons for leaving home. He did not pry, but listened intently. I never brought it up again, and neither did he. Renting my own apartment became a little too expensive, so I moved from that place a few months later. By then, I had moved ten times in twice as many years.

I settled in a small, loft, attic bedroom and shared a kitchen and bath with two guys. They were decent and respectable. It was like living with brothers. Their humorous antics kept me amused. Economically, times were tough, but I managed to find a job at the local university. Thankfully, I did not have to reveal my academic failure during the interview. No one asked to see proof of my graduation, and I certainly did not offer any. It was only a temporary position, but it was a place to start.

Unbeknownst to me, this position would provide me with the research skills I would later need to identify the root of my health problems. What was initially a temporary job would eventually become a career of years—many years, in fact. I became an expert at researching information, finding facts, and digging up resources.

Shelving away the shame of my unfinished college degree, I began working as a research assistant. One of the best things about this position was that I was surrounded by students. It was like going to work with your friends. Things were looking up; however, it was short-lived. I soon learned that I was pregnant. This could not have come at a worse time. I did not feel the joy and enthusiasm that an expectant mother would normally feel. I had major issues and fears of parenting. I had started a new job, yet was still extremely discouraged about not finishing college. I was paralyzed with fear. Then, as if the unborn child knew this, it expelled itself in a horribly painful miscarriage in the first trimester. I did not even realize what was happening—all I could feel was pain. I remember asking the doctor why I was in so much pain. He explained that I was having a miscarriage. My boyfriend, who would later become my husband, was both saddened and relieved because we were in no position to become parents. I can only remember feeling great fear for myself, for us, and for the child. I was twenty-one years old, and, although I felt confident I could take care of myself, I could not imagine how we would be able to care for a child.

The experience was a mix of sorrow and relief. In retrospect, I can understand only now what kind of stress I was experiencing at that time in my life—acute stress—the sudden, intense kind of stress. I remember leaving the hospital that day feeling very much alone. No matter what, I could not help thinking that the baby would not have wanted a mother like me anyway. I could not even get a college diploma. I thought that it was probably best that things turned out this way because it was all I could do to take care of myself. It was difficult to describe. On the one hand, I had been secretly curious and excited about the tiny life hiding inside me and could now understand why women did, in fact, become overjoyed at the news of being pregnant. On the other hand, my particular circumstances were shrouded by fear and disappointment.

The shame of being young and unmarried, the feeling of being a failure, and the fear of perpetuating the parenting style of my childhood seemed to take precedence over grief and disappointment about having lost the baby. I simply accepted the loss of my child as something that was meant to be. I did not really have time to be sad about it—I had to get over it, quick. We both did. It became something we did not discuss much. We did not have time to contemplate it—he was working long hours out of town, and I had just started a new job. This was without a doubt the lowest point in my life.

Many of my feelings I did not disclose to my friends or even my boyfriend. I did not think they would understand. To me, it seemed no matter what I did, I always had to try twice as hard as the next. Everything was an uphill battle. By this point, I was weary of it all. More than once, I entertained the thought of escaping the way I felt. I thought that, just like the baby, the world would be better off without me. I hate to admit it, but it became easy to just imagine falling asleep and never waking up. Serious thoughts poured through my mind. I know now that this was selfish of me, but back then, my mind was frantic, and my thoughts were desperate, all I could imagine was that I was a failure. Though I was raised with religion, I felt I could not even talk to God about my feelings, so I avoided him. I was convinced that once again, as in my childhood, he would only want to punish me, too. It had been so long since I had bothered with God, I could only imagine that he would not want to bother with me, either.

3

The Incurable Woman

I knew I lived a stressful life, but I figured that everyone had stress and you just had to live with it. It was not a choice for me—it was about survival. I felt like I was continuously under pressure and chronically complaining of feeling unwell. I was very young when I began my journey of diagnosis after diagnosis, spending fifteen years trying to figure out what I had actually learned long before—that if I needed anything, I would have to get it myself.

DIAGNOSIS: OVERUSE OF PAINKILLERS

When I was in high school, I developed a problem with taking pills. Not with street drugs, but pharmaceuticals. I had a leg operation when I was in tenth grade and was still living at home with my parents. After the operation, my knee was fixed, but I had started popping pills whenever I felt pain. I had actually begun raiding the medicine chest when I was a little kid, biting the childproof lids off medicine bottles. I managed to get the lids off without anyone noticing. I always complained of sore legs as far back as I could remember. No concrete diagnosis ever revealed why. The operation I had was not serious—cartilage removal in my left knee, but at fifteen, you do not want to be held up for very long. It became easy to just numb myself, once I had learned how. Throughout school, I was active in track and field and played junior women's floor hockey, but my passion was gymnastics. I loved it! It was also an escape for me. I always knew that no matter what happened, I could go out there and tumble or flip my way to happiness again. It made me feel accomplished. In my elementary years, my teammates affectionately nicknamed me "Nadia" after the famous Romanian gold-medallist. I was now on the high school team, and I did not want to have to quit. I still lived at home at this point, but I hid the fact that I took so many painkillers. No one knew, except me.

Surgery did not stop there. Again, at seventeen, I had another leg operation, after I had moved away from home. This time, it was a benign bone tumor of calcium on my left leg. This operation was a disaster. The incision was big, and the pain was terrible afterwards. It was not a serious condition, but the healing did not go well. The incision would not heal. Then it burst open and had to be taped together again. It was a really painful mess. It took a year of physiotherapy before I could bend my left leg fully again. This operation ultimately ended my many years of competitive gymnastics and sports in general. Now it was over, and I was in pain. But my consolation was that I knew I could get all the painkillers I wanted. Because of the slow healing process, I resorted to taking pills whenever I felt the slightest discomfort because this time around, I did not have time for pain to keep me down. I had to work to stay in school and could not afford to take time off. I also wanted to have some fun like the average teenager; I was dating and going out with friends, pain took up too much time and energy. Besides, I had my painkillers; they became a staple for me. So much so, that at eighteen, they affected my heart—it would pound and race. This was scary! My doctor put me on a heart monitor to determine if I had heart problems. The data from the heart monitor indicated that I did not have a heart condition, but my doctor told me I had to stop taking so many pills. At this point, I was taking a pain killer for everything and anything, but the trepidation I felt when my heart raced convinced me to take his advice. I had to wean myself off painkillers. This was not easy because I was addicted. I would not admit it then, but I know it now. As other teens might lurk in the shadows to get "street" drugs, I was a medicine cabinet junkie! I searched for painkillers, muscle relaxants, anti-inflammatories or anything that would suppress pain or bring relaxation. Eventually my sister and my boyfriend became very concerned and started to scold me whenever they saw me with a medicine bottle in my hand. My sister was forced to hide all the tablets when I lived with her, and I could only have them if the pain was unbearable. We actually got into huge fights over pills! I am convinced now that I took pills more because it became a habit than for the pain.

DIAGNOSIS: HYPOGLYCEMIA

I was also struggling with the fact that, although I was young, I felt extremely worn out. I took on temporary part time jobs in addition to my job at the university to try to whittle down my student loan. With the stress of working long hours, the disappointment of not obtaining my college diploma, and the grief of having miscarried, melancholy began to fill my days. Perhaps at this time, and at this time only, someone could have suggested to me that I was mildly depressed or feeling temporary depression.

   I eventually moved out of the loft I shared with the guys and returned to the city I had once left at age sixteen. This time, I rented a house with my younger sister and three other female roommates. It was comfortably affordable. Another positive was that it brought my younger sister and I much closer. She had been thirteen and was still living with my parents when I originally left home. At this time, she was studying in college—the college I had attended. I was in my mid-twenties and beginning to feel extremely fatigued. I would not say I was sick, but I just knew there was something wrong with the way I felt. I asked my doctor during an annual exam why I might be feeling this way. After the usual tests, he indicated that my sugar levels were somewhat low. He suggested I might be slightly hypoglycemic. I explained there was a history of diabetes in my family and asked whether I could become diabetic. He said that if I watched what I ate and continued to exercise, I should not fall victim to the hereditary pattern of Type II diabetes set by my grandmother and great grandmother.

Aware of my difficult past, he asked me how I felt emotionally. I replied that I thought I was okay, that there was nothing much I could do about the past, and that I had felt optimistic about my research job. He did not directly ask about depression, but I could tell he suspected it. He also left me thinking that hypoglycemia could be a problem. At that point, I did not know much about it and did not know that unrelenting stress could also contribute to low blood sugar. Unfortunately, the doctor did not explain any of this to me. He also did not explain that hypoglycemia could indicate chronic fatigue and was often diagnosed in a more serious condition that I will describe next. It would be years later that I would figure this out on my own.

DIAGNOSIS: CANDIDA SYNDROME

You may not know what candida is, but I imagine you know what yeast overgrowth is. The majority of women have likely experienced yeast overgrowth at least once in their lives, especially during pregnancy. Candida syndrome is an imbalance of bacteria in the body that leads to an overgrowth of fungi that often manifests itself as thrush in babies and yeast infections in adults. If you have ever had a sick baby with thrush or a yeast infection yourself, then you know what kind of suffering it can cause. Although I had suffered with symptoms of candida since roughly age thirteen, I did not know what it was until age eighteen, when a yearly physical checkup revealed this diagnosis. Usually a person can suspect a yeast infection because it most often manifests itself as the irritation with which we have become so familiar. However, with me it was much more involved than that.

I initially thought it was allergies. It would become the worst of my symptoms. It seemed ever present taking various forms and was enough to make me miserable at times. Only now do I realize the many symptoms associated with this condition. For years, I endured symptoms of food sensitivities, itching skin and rashes, (specifically on my face which was not especially visible, thankfully, but very irritating), and increased sensitivity to perfumes and cigarette smoke. This was particularly difficult when I was a waitress because the entire restaurant would fill with smoke. My eyes would burn and itch constantly in the smoke. I also experienced what seemed to feel like a "foggy" head. I had dry eyes and felt shaky and weak if I did not eat right away. I would become incredibly irritable and tired at the drop of a hat. Routinely, I was prescribed medications that seemed to help at first, only to have the symptoms return within a few weeks. I spent literally years making trips back and forth to my doctor to complain that I had been experiencing these problems and that they would not go away. Not once *did even one* doctor ever explain candida syndrome to me. They only ever gave me prescriptions and told me to avoid sugars and fatty foods.

Eventually I learned that if I indulged in sugary foods, like chocolate, it would cause further symptoms. I took every precaution not to use harsh soaps and perfumes or chemical laundry detergents. I avoided sugar as much as possible and drank gallons of cranberry juice (which I later learned is a bad thing because cranberry juice is full of sugar!). I received diagnosis after diagnosis of candida, and it seemed there was no way of making it go away. I had experienced brief relief from time to time, but nothing ever really got rid of it for good. I tried connecting it to my diet, which seemed to suggest something, but I could not figure out why I would suffer the same symptoms, even when I avoided chocolate or fatty foods. This condition was far more involved and potentially serious than I knew. Candidiasis could make you very miserable if it happened once, but experiencing it continually was beginning to make my life a living hell. At that time, there was no reason for me to relate candida to stress and fatigue; I was only ever told it was a sugar-related problem. Nevertheless, even when I avoided sugar, it would not alleviate my symptoms of candida. I was diagnosed with this condition many times throughout my teens and twenties.

DIAGNOSIS: SLEEP DISORDER—INSOMNIA

At twenty-seven my symptoms had peaked, and I began my incessant marathon of doctors' appointments. I was active, exercising, and trying to watch my weight. I was not overweight and generally did what I could to stay healthy. However, I had begun waking up in the middle of the night, 3:18 AM to be exact, and could not get back to sleep very well. I would lay there, my mind wandering all over; feeling as if I had too much energy. Eventually, around 6 a.m., I would self-exhaust and start falling back to sleep. This would have been fine, if I did not have to get up in an hour to get ready for work. Nothing sucked the life out of me worse than lack of sleep. Still, I figured it was a phase, excitement maybe, as my boyfriend—my high school sweetheart—had just proposed to me! On Christmas Day at age twenty-seven, I opened a tiny velvet box and discovered the exact engagement ring I had pined over for so long! We had dated almost steadily from age sixteen to twenty-seven, and now we were getting married! It was one thing to get married, and another thing to marry your high school sweetheart!

I thought with all the wedding planning, I just had too much going on in my head. Additionally, as a child, I had never slept well. I experienced frequent night terrors, and at times, I would sleepwalk, awakening early in the morning on the bathroom floor. It was often early enough that no one else realized that I had spent the night on the floor. I do not know why I always ended up here, perhaps the comfort and warmth of the soft, purple rug on the bathroom floor made the difference. As a child, I thought this was normal. Although my parents knew about some of my problems with sleepwalking and night terrors, I was never diagnosed with any sleep disorders. Now, I was beginning to wonder if this strange sleep pattern was resurfacing. I went back to the doctor, and he explained that I had anxiety so he gave me a mild antidepressant. I thought, I'm not depressed, I'm tired, but it seemed to help me stay asleep for a while, so I did not pay much more attention to my lack of sleep.

While planning my wedding, I felt two part-time jobs, in addition to my full-time job, were necessary to pay for it. Although my fiancé was working, it was only seasonal, and we had no financial support from our families to help with the wedding. If it was going to happen, we would have to manage it ourselves. I was burning the candle at both ends. Unable to get a decent night's sleep, I began to experience headaches. I figured it was time to find out why I was waking up so much in the night. I went back to my doctor and requested a sleep test. He agreed and sent me to a diagnostic sleep center where they hook you up like Frankenstein and tell you to go to sleep! I had all these little wires glued to my head and stuck to my arms, legs, and chest. I even had them on my eyes and nose to monitor eye movements and breathing. It was not painful or uncomfortable, but it was awkward to try to sleep in a tangle of wires.

As I spent the night at the sleep clinic, the results showed that I did in fact wake up—over forty times during the night. The most specific time recorded was around 3 AM when my test revealed an increase in alpha brain-wave activity. I later learned that alpha waves in the brain represent alertness and calm wakefulness. I was told this kind of waking was common in patients with chronic fatigue, and again they suggested that I could be depressed. I was a little surprised because this was not the first time a doctor implied that I might be depressed. I was not depressed—I was just too busy and tired. I was diagnosed with a sleep disorder because of anxiety. I was a little confused. Were they suggesting that I was depressed or that I had chronic fatigue? No one explained. Instead, my doctor prescribed a mild anti-depressant—again. I took this medication for four years until I noticed the need for more than I had initially been taking in order for it to be effective. This worried me. I had developed an addiction to prescription drugs in high school. Now, here I was, a decade later, becoming dependent on antidepressants for sleep problems. In addition, I was taking more and more of the painkillers to treat the headaches I started having.

My fear of becoming a pill-popper again drove me to a cold turkey quit. At a follow-up appointment, I told the doctor not to renew my prescription for antidepressants and that I was going to seek alternatives to deal with the pain and anxiety. I would try yoga, hot baths—whatever it took. He respected my decision. Cold turkey was a hard route to take. It was all I could do to suppress the urge to take something when I felt the symptoms that had been dragging me down for so long. I began having frequent headaches and the sleep thing was way out of control. I kept a sleep diary and logged in seven days. During the seven days, I had only slept about an hour or two each night. I felt like I was going insane. I desperately needed some sleep. Why couldn't I sleep? Why the headaches?

DIAGNOSIS: TENSION HEADACHES

The headaches I had begun to experience seemed to come shortly after my sleep disorder. These headaches would come and go, sometimes hanging around in a mild form for a few days. At other times, they would creep up on me with pounding with pain, and then suddenly it felt like I'd been hit by a train! I could not figure out why I would wake up with a headache. On occasion, my younger sister would drive me to the hospital because I could not hold my head up straight due to the pain. My eyes would water and my right eye would twitch. I was puzzled. I often took some painkillers and hoped it would subside. I saw a neurologist in the emergency room one night, and he suggested I see him in his office later that week for some tests.

I went to the appointment, had an EEG, and went through a series of neurological tests to determine if there was anything wrong in my head. I also had a CT scan. However, all the tests revealed nothing. Apparently, I was fine. No abnormality was found on my scans that could cause such headaches. Then, the doctor asked if I had experienced any depression. Again, another doctor was bringing up depression. I began to wonder if the doctors I had seen had a secret pact to convince me that I was simply depressed. I assured him I had headaches and not depression. Unfortunately, I came away with no real answers or remedies. The only option appeared to be continuing to take painkillers. The doctor's diagnosis was tension headaches.

The wedding came, and everything went wonderfully. I do not regret having to work for it. It was a beautiful summer day, and all our work and planning paid off nicely. I figured that after the wedding, the sleep deprivation and headaches would go away, and I would be fine again. I was looking forward to all the things new brides anticipate—a home, children, and perhaps even a new career. However, months went by, and my symptoms continued. I could not understand why, since I was feeling content and secure for the first time in my life.

During the first couple of years of our marriage, I focused a great deal of my attention and energy on helping my husband achieve his dream job of becoming a firefighter. After much training and commitment, we were very excited when he finally received a job offer. During the whole process, I had not worried about his choice of profession. I was also comfortable with the idea of shift work. Having lived so long on my own or with roommates, I was not someone who became anxious being alone. I was confident that he had received the best training and that he was prepared for whatever responsibilities he might encounter with this new job.

However, despite the enthusiasm we shared for his new position as a firefighter, it could not have come at a more discouraging time. His job offer came just three weeks after the terrorist attacks of September 11, 2001, after which three hundred forty-three firefighters would eventually be honored for their sacrifice that day. While the headlines announcing the tragic events of 9/11 were captivating the attention of the world, I was trying to ignore the TV images and celebrate my husband's new success. I cannot say whether this added to my stress, since we were both prepared for his commitment to becoming a firefighter; however, the timing of it all seemed to stir my emotions.

I was so proud of his achievement, but seeing the images of those who perished that day tainted the experience. When I announced his new position as a firefighter, many people asked, "Do you really want him to be a firefighter now? Look what happened in New York City." Although this would spark bits of fear in me, I was able to put it in perspective, separating the events of 9/11 from his becoming a firefighter. I knew the risks, but I also knew this was his big ambition. I was confident his superiors would guide him and resolved to entrust him to God. It was a leap of faith, but one I was willing to take. A firefighter's wife is a role itself—and one I do not regret. It has helped solidify my faith and makes me very proud every day.

Despite my enthusiasm for my husband, it did not seem to change anything about how I was feeling physically. I was not willing to suffer like this any longer. I had lived with the headaches for some time now, and they were not getting any better. I went back to the clinic, saw an on-call doctor one afternoon, and described my symptoms to her. I explained that I had gone through all kinds of tests and that they found no reason for me to have such headaches. She noted that my neck and shoulders were very tight and suggested I go for massage therapy. Having a stranger rubbing my body with warm oils was not my idea of therapy. I had always thought massage was for the hedonist. I never imagined it was useful for "real" problems, but I agreed to try it.

The doctor also referred me to yet another neurologist. I had an appointment with this neurologist, and again I completed all the neurological tests routinely performed for patients with headache complaints. The tests revealed no irregularities. They even showed me the image of my perfectly normal brain on the CT imaging screen. They explained that it is often very difficult to determine the origins of headaches. I knew this, but I had almost hoped that something would show up to explain why I had such nagging pain. The diagnosis, again, was simply headaches. I felt the headaches were worse after I had had a night or two of restless, uncomfortable sleep. If I did enjoy the odd night of sleep for more than a few hours, the headaches seemed less intense. This was also the case for my neck and shoulder stiffness. I noticed this pattern, and decided that the sleep problem and the headaches were likely related to one another. One symptom always seemed to follow another. I did not have any medical proof of this, but I did not have any proof of anything at this point.

DIAGNOSIS: TINNITUS

For as long as I could remember, I experienced an almost constant pulsing noise in my head. It was not associated with any pain; it was just annoying. It was as though I could hear my heart beating in my head. I had been hearing this sound on and off all throughout my life. I remembered being about ten years old when I first heard it, and I wondered if it was because of swimming a lot and getting water in my ears. It would come and go, and I only heard it when the sounds around me were low enough not to drown it out. I was curious about it, but I usually blocked it out or ignored it. It seemed to be worse since I had begun not sleeping well. I wondered if it was connected to my terrible headaches.

My doctor recommended a specialist. He sent me to one who performed a series of hearing tests on me. The results were normal and showed no apparent damage to my ears. He could not figure out why I had this sound in my head, but suspected it was tinnitus, so he referred me to another specialist at a larger, more advanced hearing clinic. At that appointment, the hearing specialist also performed several hearing tests and concluded that there was nothing wrong with my hearing nor did I have any problems with the mechanics of my ears. He looked at me, observing the dark circles under my eyes, and suggested I was anemic. I did not know what that had to do with my hearing. Then, he asked me if I was depressed. I almost punched him! Why were doctors suggesting again, that I could be depressed? I assured him I was not depressed. He looked back at me skeptically.

Why were these doctors suggesting depression every time I asked them what was wrong with me? Was everyone with "mystery symptoms" being diagnosed as depressed? I explained that I had not been sleeping very well. He ruled out that the tinnitus was caused by the usual culprits like being exposed to loud sounds or some kind of injury or blockage. He ordered MRI tests for my head to rule out any blockage of arteries that could be causing the pulsing sound I was hearing. I also had a Doppler test to determine if there were any arterial blockages. The tests revealed nothing that would clearly cause tinnitus. Yet, he did conclude that with the muscle tension and stiffness in my shoulders and neck, that I likely had pulsatile tinnitus from tension. There was nothing more he could do except an angiogram. However, he cautioned this was far too risky for something that was not causing pain. It was irritating, but not painful. I did not want an angiogram. I did not like the idea of inserting a tube into an artery in my leg and running it up to my brain. I agreed that it was too risky and left with a diagnosis of pulsatile tinnitus.

There was nothing more I could do. I remained frustrated. Why did I have a bothersome sound in my head? Maybe I was hearing things and going a little crazy. Although all the tests were normal, I could not help wondering if I was imagining all this. Perhaps my symptoms were psychosomatic, and this was depression after all. Was this what depression is? Is it a bunch of sneaky symptoms that are seemingly impossible to diagnose? How could a sound in my head, like the pulsing of tinnitus, imply depression? I wished someone else could hear what I could hear. Then, perhaps, doctors would consider something other than depression.

One morning as I lay in bed, my husband lay with his head close to me. Suddenly, he leaned over, put his ear up against mine, and told me to be very quiet. He said he could hear a "swishing sound" when he put his ear close against mine. *He* could hear the sound that I could hear that pulsed with my heartbeat! I was elated! Someone else could hear what I had been hearing for so long. It felt like a confirmation that I was not crazy or depressed. Yet, I felt I had no choice but to live with it…for now.

I was getting too many diagnoses and too few answers. I wondered how anyone could live a happy life with all these symptoms at once. The only way I could control the headaches was with painkillers. The only way I could regulate my sleep was with antidepressants. The only way to neutralize the candida was with ineffective over the counter prescriptions. And there was no way to eliminate the pulsing sounds in my head.

It was like a vicious cycle with no end in sight. The symptoms persisted and drove me crazy. I would cry to my husband, my sisters, and even my mom—telling them that I could not stand this anymore. It was too much to swallow. I recall sobbing in the middle of the night because I was so tired, yet I could not sleep. I remember having to pull over to the side of the road and wait for the pain in my head to subside. The pulsing, swishing sound in my head continued. My neck and shoulders burned with pain and tension, and *Candida* built a permanent home in my body! Why was I feeling this way? Every test was negative. According to the doctors, I was "perfectly normal." Maybe it *was* "all in my head." I began to wonder. Was I becoming a hypochondriac? Were my problems psychosomatic? Was I really depressed?

My doctor pretty much had a chair in the waiting room with my name on it. Regardless of what the tests showed, there was something not right in my body. It was making me feel terrible, and I seriously began to believe that in fact, I was depressed. I just could not figure out why I would be so depressed. My life was fine now: I was reasonably healthy (I thought); I was happily married; and I had a decent job. I simply could not pinpoint anything that would validate a diagnosis of depression. I did not want to accept this. It was so frustrating because it seemed the doctors did not believe me. No one could tell me what was robbing me of my energy and health. Frustration grew into anger. I became angry enough to try to figure this elusive thing out on my own. It strengthened my resolve that I was not going to suffer like this anymore.

4

Chronic Stress—Depression's Evil Twin!

Stressed? Worried? Anxious? My sister once told me she felt like "a tick about to pop." I laughed, realizing she was right. That is life, a constant process of action and reaction. Unfortunately, we seem to be more in action than ever before. As technology advances, so do we. The advances in technology do not seem to have allowed us to slow down as promised. Instead, modern technology appears to have increased our workload and complicated our lifestyles in ways we did not expect. We seem to have less time than ever before. Time has become precious. Regardless of what we do, it just keeps going. There is no way to stop the clock or hold on to the sun just a few hours longer. This seems especially true for women. It was also the case with me. Women seem more stressed out today than ever before. Juggling a career alongside the roles of wife and/or motherhood require women to stretch their day—unrealistically.

Most women find themselves looking for a twenty-fifth hour in a twenty-four-hour day. If only we could buy that twenty-fifth hour! What would we do with it? Would we find something else to clean, to cook, or another phone call to make? Would we wash another load of laundry or catch up on paperwork at the office? Or, would we sit and read that book we hadn't cracked open yet, run a nice, hot bath, or suit up and head to the gym? What would you do with an extra hour? The way I had been living; it would have just been another hour of work. The only way to control time is to control ourselves. This can be hard for women because of their maternal drive. Because women are caregivers by nature, we tend to sacrifice for our spouses, partners, children, family and friends. It is our nature.

However, it is easy to see how women are pushing themselves to the limit, burning the candle at both ends, and ultimately, suffering for it. Many women feel the need to be Superwomen! Just go to a store and view the plethora of popular books and magazines for women, if you need proof. You'll see dozens of headlines for reducing stress. Advertisements rhyme off solutions and cures that could rival any Dr. Seuss book! All the best ways for reducing stress. You see miracle makeovers, fat busters, and thigh burners. There are diet tips and low fat dips; ten-minute dinners and fast tummy trimmers; twelve ways to great shape and to find a hot mate; the world's greatest spas, and how to beat the blahs. We are told how to be rich, sexy, and thin, and not to eat chocolate because it's a sin!

Advertisements and societal expectations pressure women to succeed at it all. I do not mean the expected stressors of planning a wedding, getting a new job, or losing a friend. I mean the almost unrelenting stress of daily life. When all is said and done, understanding the effects of daily stress and of life in the fast lane is something most women do not have time to think about. I know I did not seriously consider it. But when my symptoms became so severe, what choice did I have? For me, it was a choice to passively accept my condition or take the road less traveled. I decided I would find my own way to better health and a better understanding of stress—even if it were the last thing I did!

SEEK AND YE SHALL FIND

I am a research assistant for a living. Much of my job involves finding information. Often the information is hard to find or I only have a vague description of what they need and have to dig from there. I knew how to find books, articles, news publications—you name it. I knew my way around a library like my own backyard. I was specifically skilled at finding information on the Internet. Naturally, I decided to put my skills to work for my own health. I began to search my symptoms, one by one, and began to understand more and more about each one. I focused on my sleep problem, suspecting that all my symptoms could be related to poor sleep. Through this research, I came to understand the importance of sleep and the effects of sleep deprivation. Sleep was more important than I had ever realized. It restored the body in a way no medicine or therapy ever could. After researching sleep, I was motivated to control the problem.

It had been two years since my last sleep test, and I decided I wanted it done again, but more thoroughly. I searched in my area for a doctor who specialized in sleep disorders. I found one, got the referral from my regular doctor, and had a sleep test done again. This test required that I keep a sleep diary for two weeks before my actual sleep test in the lab. I kept the diary—recording every activity including sleeping patterns. I did not sleep much, but it was good to record it. Also, the doctor gave me a multi-paged questionnaire regarding my general health, diet, job, family, and my sleep patterns throughout childhood up until the present. There were also several pages asking questions that I eventually realized were supposed to determine my psychological status.

I hoped no one would again suggest I was depressed. Depression seemed the easiest route for doctors to explain what was wrong with me and suggest that it was "all in my head." I believe depression exists as a real illness, yet I felt this was not my problem because what I was feeling was mostly physical. Although I had experienced a great deal of disappointment in my life, I remained positive and carried an almost limitless sense of hope. I had *hoped* my way through many crises and never felt hopeless, even at my lowest.

Something made me try again; something kept me going. I knew that other women who had experienced similar symptoms were also told that depression was the culprit or that it was "all in their heads." Yet, I could not accept that we are all just depressed. It seems to be a widely accepted diagnosis, but is it always a correct diagnosis? Everyone can experience mood swings and emotional sways on a daily basis and still be in good health. It was too easy to prescribe anti-depressants. I did not want to fall victim to a nation cruising on Prozac. I was well aware of the statistics on this. Maybe it was helping some people lead normal lives. Being placed on anti-depressants certainly helped me to sleep better by shutting down my brain, but I felt it was only a pacifier.

I had developed too much dependency on prescriptions all my life. I did not want to depend on medicine to sustain my life and make me "feel" better. Rather than attempt a "neurological makeover" with more drugs, I wanted to be better-period! I noticed how sleep deprivation and muscle tension could be related to each other, and I could even add headaches into the equation due to lack of restorative sleep; but what about candida syndrome, hypoglycemia, and tinnitus? Where did these fit in?

I went for a second sleep diagnostic test. In the morning, two doctors completed my consultation. One doctor was a sleep disorder specialist, and the other was a neurologist. They mutually agreed that I had a sleep disorder. Their diagnosis was middle insomnia. I did not know insomnia came in sections. Middle insomnia means waking in the middle of sleeping—around 3:00-4:00 AM, which I did routinely.

They proceeded with their analysis, explaining to me that I was "hyper-vigilant." I had never heard that term before. It sounded like something from an action movie. The doctors explained it in terms of the "fight or flight" stress response. I had heard of this before. Apparently, I was someone in "fight mode," which is a normal reaction to stress, except that you are not supposed to function like this on a daily basis. I responded with a hesitant laugh, mixed with a tone of agreement. I suspected that I must have been in this mode since age sixteen, maybe even earlier. I felt as though I was fighting all the time, especially when I was supposed to be relaxed or asleep. Could I be fighting in my sleep as I was fighting when awake? The doctor who analyzed my sleep test described my problem as he saw it: like a soldier on a battlefield.

STILL AT WAR

These doctors explained the term hyper-vigilance to me using the analogy of a returning soldier who had "not yet realized he didn't have to fight anymore," someone who remained ready to fight at any moment. My sleep test results revealed as much brain wave activity at night as would normally represent alert wakefulness. I was like a soldier, camouflaged, waiting to defend. This was their descriptive analogy of how I had been living. Hyper is described as excessive or exaggerated, and vigilance is noted as being alert, keenly watchful, and able to detect trouble or danger.[1] Thus, they began describing the condition of post-traumatic stress disorder. People often use this term to describe the stress that Vietnam veterans suffered after returning home from war. Many of these soldiers returned home only to end up in lives of crime and turmoil, sometimes ended by suicide. Often the soldier's "flight" mechanism was to act out the violence and trauma they witnessed and experienced during the war. Post-traumatic stress disorder can occur after experiencing life-threatening events, enduring episodes of trauma, or witnessing horrific events. People who suffer from this disorder usually relive the events through nightmares and flashbacks.[2] Hyper-vigilance, on the other hand, is more of a pre-post traumatic stress disorder. Some have suggested that many of the soldiers who had come home were "still at war," even though the war had ended. Many were in a constant state of hyper-vigilance. Based on my sleep test results and my consultation, the doctors concluded that I had been in this state of hyper-vigilance for quite some time. After explaining this, one of the doctors looked at me matter-of-factly, and asked calmly, "So, what are you fighting?"

He hit a nerve in me with that question. For once, I let my guard down and accepted this description. I knew he was describing exactly how I had lived for as long as I could remember. The question was almost haunting. Honestly, I had not lived; I had only been surviving. I had come to expect that I could only rely on myself. Generally, I trusted no one else, even though I was happily married and my life was much more secure than it had ever been. I had convinced myself for years that I would only ever be able to count on myself. I sat in that office chair and felt like he was talking to someone who had lived many more years than the calendar was saying. That moment, when the doctor looked square at me and asked what I had been fighting, was the first time I realized I had always been prepared to fight should something attempt to sabotage my efforts. I expected the unexpected and was armed and ready for the worst of times, even if they turned out good. It is how I learned to survive. But was that a healthy way to live?

I explained how I had developed an attitude of self-reliance because I had trouble trusting anyone else. I explained my childhood, my decision to leave home at a young age, and my feelings of failure. I told him no matter how hard I tried, my ship had not come in yet. I was still on the dock waiting, I guess. He asked me what kept me waiting. I said it was because I had never stopped hoping. I was not someone who despaired to the point of hopelessness. I had always kept going with a sense that things would get better and, eventually, be fine. After I explained this to the doctors, they assured me I was definitely not depressed in any clinical sense. Based on my tests and testimony, they concluded that I did not show signs of clinical depression. They did agree, however, that I had lived a very stressful life and that this was playing a large role in the way I was feeling. They suggested therapy to help me deal with hyper-vigilance. In addition, they prescribed a short-acting hypnotic to be used only when I awoke at night. If I could manage this problem, I could get the restorative sleep my body needed. They felt the drugs would help me return to sleep and not give me a feeling of drowsiness or hangover in the morning. However, when I took them, I experienced daytime headaches and drowsiness. Because of my addictive tendencies, I proceeded cautiously as far as taking more prescription drugs.

Chronic stress is like depression's evil twin. It produces many of the same symptoms and resembles depression, but medically they are two different things. Chronic stress can often lead to depression, and knowing this, I was determined to avoid it! I left my appointment feeling relieved. Finally, the doctors were not telling me I was depressed or even that I could be depressed. Although they did explain my sleep disorder, I still felt I was carrying around the many symptoms that had spun me in this crazy circle of diagnoses. Although they had not implied another diagnosis of depression, I was still not satisfied with all the results. This is not to suggest that the doctors were not doing their jobs. It seemed the only way to treat each of these symptoms was with drugs. Unfortunately, these drugs often required more drugs to combat their side effects.

I began wondering if I was sub-clinically sick with something that doctors traditionally do not look for. What else could be going on inside my body that could cause me to feel this way and was so hard to detect? I tried to identify a pattern to my problems. I started keeping track of what I felt and when I felt it. I began to suspect that all of my symptoms were connected to the same problem, but I did not know where to begin with this hypothesis. Once I had explained some of my problems to a co-worker who told me her husband once had sleep trouble and had found great relief after seeing a naturopath. I did not like the sound of this. The idea of naturopathic doctors had always formed an image in my mind of old, bearded, tree-huggers who boiled roots and made poultices out of gross things to treat weird people who believed in that "natural" stuff. I envisioned some crazy "witchdoctor" experimenting with mythical cure-alls on me. I now realize that this was a much-distorted view of natural medicine. In any case, I was desperate and at the end of my rope. I was ready to eat weeds, drink boiled bark, or pack a poultice if it helped. If it did not work, I was running out of ideas. I made an appointment and had my first visit with a naturopath.

Not surprisingly, this visit was different from any other doctor I had seen. The doctor listened intently for quite some time as I explained my grocery list of symptoms. She wrote it all down. After I had explained my symptoms, she began to question me about my family, job, diet, activities, relationships, and even my sleep patterns in childhood. She seemed to be examining me from a historical point of view and comparing it to my current symptoms. She explained that my body was responding to a great deal of stress, from current stresses to past ones. I explained that I made many resolutions about my life and that I had made peace with the mistakes and hard times I had lived through. I told her my life was much better now.

However, she suggested that even though, perhaps, my mind had resolved things, my body had not caught up with my mind yet. She felt that prolonged emotional stress had built up even though I was mentally okay. Emotional stress manifested itself physically, and it was taking its toll on me. She implied that I was wounded though I had not stopped long enough to realize this. This doctor made me realize that I was not just stressed out sometimes, but rather chronically, and had been for a very long time.

She encouraged me to learn more about health and stress. I began to look at stress more closely. I would pinpoint certain instances when I felt as bad as my circumstances. I could identify patterns in my life that correlated to my health problems. I worked with the naturopath in determining how stress was affecting my health. I followed her advice to try to recognize symptoms when they occurred, rather than impatiently doing whatever it took to rid myself of them. I kept a diet journal and paid very close attention to my sleep patterns and headaches. I began to regularly monitor my use of prescription drugs. I became acutely aware of when I felt symptoms of sleeplessness, headaches, or food cravings. I was learning to dig deeper—to look beyond my symptoms to see the root of my health problems. When I did this, I concluded that everything was beginning to point in the same direction, to chronic stress.

UNDERSTANDING STRESS

Stress is a complex phenomenon. What stress is to some, may not be the same for another. What might make one person freak out might not make another even flinch. Stress depends on the individual. Though popular media advertisements may have you believe otherwise, it is impossible to be stress-free. To be completely free of stress would ultimately mean death.³ Moreover, it is not so much what causes the stress as it is how you chose to react to it. This was a major shift in thinking for me. I read and researched until I saturated myself with information about all of the symptoms I had been experiencing for so long. Although I could relate them to one another under the term stress, how could stress be defined in the body? What was happening to my body when I experienced stress?

I started to think of my body as a machine—the mechanics, the physical structure, and the nervous system (like the electrical system). Throughout my search, I was led to areas of neurology, internal medicine, and immunology that I had no idea existed. I was fascinated by what I was reading, but much of it was very technical and advanced so that there was little that I could actually understand. I tried to piece things together and imagined what else I was made up of—bones, muscles—the biology of it all. But what else could be orchestrating the way I was feeling? I was missing something until I began to think about chemistry—the blood, the fluids, the hormones and the…wait a minute—hormones? What was their role? Did they have anything to do with stress?

I found a great deal of information on hormones and the glandular system. Pulling at straws, I thought my problems could be related to my thyroid since it was a gland and it secreted hormones. I explored this area and even had a thyroid test. I learned that with a thyroid disorder you could feel lethargic, lack concentration, have poor sleep, and have difficulty losing weight, and even experience mood swings and symptoms of depression. That had to be it, I thought. The thyroid plays a major role in controlling our metabolism, and hypothyroidism, an under-active thyroid, can certainly cause all of these symptoms and more.⁴ However, my thyroid test came back completely normal. I became so frustrated that I am sure it made my symptoms worse, but it also made me persevere. Were there other hormones I did not know about, and if so, where were they coming from? What did they have to do with stress? I sat at my computer, wracking my brain, as I typed the words "stress hormones" into my search engine. I had no idea what I was looking for because I had never heard of such a thing as stress hormones. I anticipated with a glimmer of hope that I would find something.

Finally, I struck gold!

I stumbled upon endocrinology—the very intriguing study of the glandular system that secretes hormones into the blood and lymph system. Here I would begin to understand the hormonal response to stress and come across a word I had never heard before, but that would become very important to my understanding of stress and its effects on the body—my body! The word was *cortisol*. What I eventually discovered about stress and hormones, specifically cortisol, was the first step I would take in seriously changing my lifestyle, which was essential to my health and well being.

CORTISOL: THE MYSTERY HORMONE

The entire hormonal system reacts very strongly to stress. I already knew about hormones like estrogen, progesterone, adrenaline, and even, epinephrine. I knew some of the functions of these hormones in the body, particularly estrogen, but I had never heard of cortisol. I had no idea what it was or that it even existed in the body. I knew of cortisone for treatment of allergies, and that was about it. I found a great deal of information about hormones in general, but when it came to cortisol, there was precious little in the easy reading section. I decided to do some more research; after all, I had excellent skills for finding this kind of information. Through scientific journals and articles, I found some useful things. One summary stood out particularly well and prompted more research on this stress hormone.

In the journal *Psychoneuroendocrinology* (not your typical leisurely reading), I read a paper by Alfred T. Sapse that summarized cortisol and it's relationship to disease as follows:

> Elevated cortisol is found in many diseases, including infectious, age-related, depression and depression-associated conditions; even in some with no known origin. While it was initially thought that "high cortisol" is the result of these diseases, there is mounting evidence to the contrary, namely, that high cortisol actually plays a major role in inducing them.[5]

I definitely could relate to the phrase "no known origin." It felt like all my symptoms had no known origin. I read more articles about cortisol and its ability to create all kinds of symptoms and problems in the body that could potentially be hard to diagnose.

However, unless you're an avid reader of medical journals, you're not likely to discover these things in plain, easy-to-understand terms. Although there is much information about hormones and how they affect us, particularly women, it was difficult to find information about stress hormones, specifically cortisol. Unless you were a doctor of some kind, you were not likely to refer to stress in terms of a hormonal response. You hear people referring to stress all the time in language like frazzled and basket case, but you never hear anyone saying, "My stress hormones are out of control!" Not many people really seem to know about cortisol, yet many researchers refer to as the "top gun of all stress hormones."[6] I finally discovered that cortisol could contribute to many of the symptoms I had been suffering from.

Hormones play a larger role in our health than most of us are even aware. When hormones are out of balance, they can produce serious health problems. I had no idea that imbalanced stress hormones, particularly cortisol, could produce such negative effects on my health. I figured hormones provoked irritable teenagers or just hung out in your body, showing up now and then to let you know you were getting older! Now, I wanted to know everything about stress hormones, especially cortisol. First, I decided to have my own cortisol levels checked—something I did not know I could do, until now.

When I asked my doctor to check my cortisol levels, he looked at me as if I had asked him to perform a lobotomy! I told him I had been researching a great deal about this hormone and felt it was playing a huge part in my health problems. He replied, "You're talking about endocrinology here," (as if to imply I was in way over my head), to which I responded, "Yes, I know that." He assured me, as if on cue, that my cortisol levels should be fine. Regardless, I insisted on the test. He eventually agreed, but seemed both surprised by and somewhat skeptical of my assumption. Perhaps it seemed I was in way over my head, but I knew my health history.

I knew I had made a connection in my research to cortisol, stress, and my health. I was the one who was experiencing sleep disturbance, headaches, and candida. I knew I felt chronically fatigued and that the pain in my neck and shoulders was not "all in my head." I knew I had gained weight, specifically in my lower abdominal area, even though I was exercising. I was only thirty-two, but physically, I felt like someone twice my age. I felt like I was dragging each day behind me like a heap of rocks! I still had my whole life ahead of me; I had ambitions, dreams, and hopes for a family. I could no longer afford to be wandering aimlessly from doctor to doctor, feeling like a total hypochondriac.

A week later, I had a cortisol test. I learned that cortisol could be measured in blood, urine, or saliva. Mine was checked in my fasting blood. The test was performed in the morning and again in the afternoon of the same day. The results indicated my cortisol level to be two times higher than normal in the morning and three times higher than normal in the afternoon. The doctor was perplexed and said that he spoke with a colleague (an endocrinologist) who suggested I have the test done again to verify the results. A week later, my cortisol levels were just as high as the last test in both the morning and afternoon readings. I then returned for a follow-up consultation with the doctor to discuss these findings. He looked at me matter-of-factly, and said, "You were right about your cortisol."

So…What Is Cortisol?

One of a number of chemical messengers (hormones) in the body, cortisol is a steroid hormone secreted by the adrenal glands. Cortisol is actually made in our body from cholesterol (not the bad kind we are urged to avoid, but the good kind—there is a good kind).[7] It functions in our brain with something called circadian rhythm. Circadian rhythm is like the clock in our brain, which controls our sleep-wake pattern.[8] Cortisol is the primary stress hormone, and our bodies require it in order to function smoothly. It is one of two types of hormones referred to as adaptive hormones. The adaptive hormones are the anti-inflammatory and pro-inflammatory hormones. The anti-inflammatory hormones are also called glucocorticoids (cortisol belongs to this group). Their function is to "inhibit excessive defensive reactions." The pro-inflammatory hormones, also called mineralcorticoids, "stimulate defense reactions."[9] If we have too much or too little cortisol, it can lead to a variety of symptoms and diseases.

When the body reacts to stress, stress hormones are released throughout the entire body, rather than go to one specific area where the stress is localized.[10] Cortisol regulates blood pressure and cardiovascular function, as well as how our body uses protein, carbohydrate, and fat. When we experience any kind of stress, either physical or psychological, cortisol secretion increases. Many other factors including drugs, pregnancy, intense exercise, and even diet, can raise cortisol levels.[11] At this point, however, I was really only interested in how chronic stress could increase cortisol levels.

Through research, I was able to understand how chronic stress operated in me. I realized there was so much I did not know about my own body and health. I was determined to find out what was wrong and fix it. I needed to break this vicious cycle and live a normal, healthy life. With the help of my doctor, the naturopath, and my own research, I learned how the body works during stress. Stress and its effects could manifest themselves in many different ways; however, identifying stress as the root of the problem was only half the work. I did not realize that prolonged stress—living in "fight or flight" mode—could have such an effect on your health. I wondered why it was so hard to pinpoint what was wrong with me.

Why had it taken so long to put all my symptoms together and identify chronic stress as being a main contributor? Likely, it is because I was so caught up with treating the symptoms, that I paid little attention to the root problem. Though the symptoms I had were not serious enough to warrant hospitalization, I realize their potential severity. Symptoms were the way in which my body was trying to tell me that something was wrong. I was not clinically "sick" or even generally sick by any testing standards. However, I was sick, just not sick enough to warrant the attention that other diseases might require. My ambiguous condition certainly frustrated me—maybe that is why the doctors often suggested depression and other psychological diagnoses. However, if I had not persisted in finding a reason for my poor health, chronic stress could have easily led to a diagnosis of clinical depression and who knows what else!

To be completely satisfied, I had the levels of various other hormones in my body checked. They assessed estrogen, progesterone, testosterone, prolactin and DHEA. DHEA (dehydroepiandrosterone) is an immune-enhancing and anti-aging hormone. Call it the "fountain of youth" hormone. It is what keeps us young; however, as we age, DHEA decreases. (I thought this one might show up indicating I was well beyond my true age!) If this hormone is low, it can also cause various problems. These other hormone levels all tested normal in my body. The only one out of control was cortisol. My doctor then decided to do a test that would determine if my brain was able to recognize when my body was releasing too much cortisol. Administering a synthetic glucocorticoid, called dexamethasone, does the trick. When the body receives the synthetic glucocorticoid, the brain normally detects the increase in glucocorticoid secretion by the adrenals and responds by sending out something called corticotrophin releasing factor (CRF)—a signal back to the adrenals to reduce glucocorticoid (cortisol) secretion. However, if the brain fails to respond to the dexamethasone (increase in glucocorticoids), then it continues to pump out CRF. It is described as "dexamethasone resistance" and is often present in patients with depression.[12]

The results of my dexamethasone test revealed that my brain did in fact respond to the influx of the synthetic hormones, and when they checked my cortisol level again, this time it measured at normal levels. What a relief! I had often wondered if there was something not right in my head and began to believe I was clinically depressed. This test revealed that my brain was responding properly. However, cortisol was still the problem, as the dexamethasone only suppressed cortisol for a short while—maybe for the rest of the day, and that was it. I still had to figure out how to reduce my cortisol levels, and this became the focus of my investigation.

Until now, I had taken much of my life and age for granted. I figured that I was too young to have experienced the effects of chronic stress, so I did not worry about it much. Interestingly, my research revealed I was not alone. I read the results of a survey by the Heart and Stroke Foundation of Canada in February 2000, in which 53 percent of respondents stated that time pressures contributed to their stress levels. The report indicated that Canadians felt that there were "simply not enough hours in the day to do all they needed or wanted to do." The statistics also showed that 43 percent, almost half, of adults over the age of thirty are stressed by factors such as jobs, family, and finances. Almost 30 percent reported that they had lost valuable sleep because of stress.

However, I was alarmed to learn that almost 75 percent of the respondents coped with their stress by watching TV, eating comfort foods (like refined sugars and carbohydrates), smoking cigarettes, or drinking alcohol; furthermore, those under more frequent stress reported eating even more fast food and smoking more cigarettes. These lifestyle habits debilitate our health. The report concludes by advising readers to "become familiar with your personal warning signs of stress" and identify how it is affecting you.[13]

With stress contributing so much to disease, it was becoming clear to me that statistics like this were much more serious than I imagined. Research has concluded stress is the main cause of almost 80 percent of illnesses—serious diseases like heart disease, psychological disorders, cancer, and hormonal dysfunctions.[14] It was this hormone connection that so interested me. Because we cannot easily measure the damage caused by stress, it is somewhat of a paradox in that the physiological response of the body to stress is two-fold; it protects and restores, yet has the ability to destroy.[15]

Acute stress usually invokes a response and then subsides. However, chronic stress is more cumulative and persistent. It is defined by feelings of tiredness, fatigue, anger, irritability and lack of energy.[16] In *The End of Stress As We Know It*, by Dr. Bruce McEwen and Elizabeth Norton Lasley, Dr. McEwen sums up the negative effects of a system originally designed to protect us. He states, "although stress in the sense of challenging events is inevitable to some degree, being stressed-out is not. It is not inevitable or normal for the very system designed to protect us to become a threat in itself." [17]

There was no way I was going to be a statistic! I felt I had to do something quick. I asked my doctor if there was anything that could reduce cortisol levels. He indicated there was no successful drug treatment aimed specifically at reducing high cortisol levels. Instead, he said that only by prescribing anti-depressant medication could I get some relief from the stress. Again, this was just masking the problem—it was not fixing it. It was up to me to get things back in order. However, with no drug treatment available (not that I really wanted to take any more prescriptions anyway) and so little information about cortisol for the layperson, I knew that my next move was to research as much as I could about reducing excess cortisol.

WHO KNEW?

If stress hormones, like cortisol made up such an important part of our health and well being, then why had I never heard anything about this? Perhaps one reason could be that topics like estrogen and hormone replacement therapy have dominated women's health issues. Cortisol, however, seems very much a mystery unless you are specifically seeking it out. I wanted to find out what my peers knew about cortisol—if anything. I decided to do my own little experiment. This was not going to be a major scientific study or anything, but I figured some general survey questions about cortisol and stress would help me understand the knowledge of others. While I did this for my own information, I think the results would be beneficial to share.

My research group consisted of forty women, ranging in age from nineteen to fifty-seven and living in Canada and the United States. I used this group to take a survey. I asked first, how old they were. Then I asked if they had ever heard of cortisol and if they knew what it was. Afterward, I asked them a question to see what they preferred—time or money (these were the two most common "stressors" because people seemed to refer to these more than anything else). Finally, I asked them to tell me how they would rate their stress levels on a daily basis, not just during stressful events, but *regularly*. I used a scale of one to ten (one being very low, five being average, and ten being extreme).

My results were rather surprising. The replies showed that 75 percent of the women had no idea what cortisol was and only 40 percent had ever even heard the word. Of those replies, most did not even know that it was a hormone! Only 1 percent replied they knew exactly what it was. Concerning the two stressors, half the women answered that time was of equal value to them as money. This especially surprised me because I would have thought most people would naturally prefer money. The most disturbing result was that 80 percent reported that they felt their average daily stress levels were above moderate (above five). These results amazed me. It meant that many women, as many as 80 percent in this study, reported higher than average stress on a daily basis and yet three-quarters of them had no idea what cortisol was.

If high cortisol was a factor in how I was feeling, then could stress hormones be making others feel the same way? Could elevated stress hormones be a major contributor to common health problems, and if so, why was there so little information available to describe the process of stress and stress hormones in the body? I felt that if I understood the process of stress in my body, then perhaps I would have been able to cope better. I knew I had chronic stress, but I did not know it could make me feel as badly as I had felt for many years.

What I found so interesting from my research is that there is a real effect happening inside me during stressful times. It made sense that my poor health was likely connected to my high-stress lifestyle. I was never convinced of depression, but I was completely convinced that high levels of stress (and stress hormones) were the basis of my illness. I could trace the path of chronic stress in my life and how it could be linked to insomnia, headaches, fatigue, pain, and possibly candida, although at this point, I could not figure out how candida fit into the equation.

5

Going to the Root of the Problem

Everybody has it, everybody talks about it, yet few people have taken the trouble to find out what stress really is.

—Hans Selye

DISSECTING STRESS AND DISTRESS

The Canadian physician and endocrinologist, Dr. Hans Selye once said, "Man should not try to avoid stress any more than he would shun food, love or exercise."[1] When I first read this statement, I thought this guy was nothing more than a mad scientist! Who on earth would invite or even entertain stress? Then I read more and understood Dr. Selye's insights from his lifelong study of stress. Selye defined stress as, "the non-specific response of the body to any demand."[2] He was right when he said non-specific. Dr. Selye spent fifty years studying the causes and effects of stress. He discovered that "patients who had a variety of health complaints had many of the same symptoms, which he attributed to their bodies' efforts to respond to stress."[3] Selye indicates that stress is not just tension, nervousness, or even the result of something damaging.

Stress is essentially anything that places a demand on our body.[4] He states: "no matter what you do, or what happens to you, there arises a demand for the necessary energy required to maintain life, resist aggression, and constantly adapt to external influences."[5] Even when we are at rest or sleeping, we are experiencing stress in the body, as the organs keep working, the brain keeps functioning, and it takes energy to even remain breathing. Both tragedy and triumph, therefore, can be considered as stress because both elicit a response from the body. The stressors can be different, but both require a biological response.[6] Selye claims, "it is not the stress that harms us but rather, *distress*—the prolonged emotional stress that we don't deal with properly."[7]

He concludes that the majority of us do not even realize that there is a difference between stress and distress.[8]

I brought this concept to the women's research group I studied and asked specifically what they would want to know about stress. Almost every one replied they wanted to know how to avoid stress. Their answers did not indicate they understood there was a difference between stress and distress. Keeping Selye's view in mind that to avoid stress or be stress-free would be impossible, I understood that what these women were really saying was they wanted to know how to avoid the negative aspects of stress—the distress.

Because stress itself is not necessarily negative, it makes it very difficult to understand. However, distress is more straightforward. It is defined as anything that causes pain, anxiety, strain, or sorrow.[9] Distress is the harmful side of stress. Selye discovered that stress had a direct affect on three main areas of the body—the immune system, the hormonal system, and the digestive system.[10] These were the three areas in which many of my symptoms showed up. When we think of stress, we usually think of it in a negative light, which we learn to associate with discomfort, anxiety, or weariness about something. However, Selye states: "it is immaterial whether the agent or situation we face is pleasant or unpleasant" as any demand upon the body, be it joyful or sorrowful, requires bodily adaptation.[11]

It might be helpful to think of the body as analogous to a brand new car—right out of the factory. If you had the car delivered to your home, parked it in a warm, dry garage and never drove it, never even started it, in 10 years, it would still be like brand new—untouched and mechanically sound. It would never have experienced work. It would have had no demand placed on it, no stress applied to it. However, once it leaves the garage and drives anywhere, even in the most ideal conditions, it will experience wear and tear. Unless we maintain the car, it will wear out and break down. Even if we give the best care to maintain that car, it will still sustain regular wear and tear. If not properly maintained, it will eventually break down. The same is true with our bodies.

Too much stress or distress (negative stress) can contribute to an entire alphabet of disorders and diseases. I learned that there are two types of stress, acute and chronic. Acute stress occurs when circumstances cause us to react quickly. Again, stress is a daily thing. Simply lifting weights or running to catch the bus can generate stress. These experiences are not burdensome; they could even be exciting things, like planning a wedding or a holiday. Hence, I felt stressed when planning my wedding because I knew I would have so many things to do to get ready for the big day, even though it was a very exciting and happy time. Acute stress is typically short-term and can be a good thing because it challenges us and gives us strength to achieve our goals.[12]

Chronic stress is different. It is like being in a continuous state of unease. It normally causes muscle tension, stiffness, shallow breathing, and a constant surge of stress hormones pumping through your body. This interferes with other body functions and often results in compromised health and illness.[13] It was the kind of stress I was familiar with. Only, I was not looking at the stress, I was feeling its symptoms. Instead of dealing with the stress, I was feeling the effects of distress. Chronic stress can manifest itself in many forms including physical, mental, emotional, chemical, nutritional, traumatic, and psycho-spiritual. A constant and unrelenting negative in any of these areas is chronic stress. Chronic stress also causes immune system suppression, which over time can cause disease in our bodies.[14]

Acute stress can also make us sick, but is often associated with something positive, like starting a new job. However, chronic stress is always bad. It is the kind of stress you cannot escape. When we experience stress, a whole process happens in the area of the brain called the hypothalamus. The hypothalamus is a major command centre that signals hormonal releases to control bodily functions like temperature, blood pressure, heartbeat, carbohydrate and fat metabolism, and blood sugar levels. It is also jointly involved in regulating our sleep-wake cycles.[15] In simple terms, a hormone is released in this area of the brain to race ahead and tell the pituitary gland (again, in our head) to send yet another hormone signal to the adrenal glands (near our kidneys) to start pumping out hormones (glucocorticoids, including cortisol) during times of stress. The path that stress follows in the body is often referred to as the HPA Axis, or the hypothalamic-pituitary-adrenal axis. Therefore, a great deal of stress is not only figuratively "all in our head," but it is also literally all in our head! Chronic stress keeps cortisol levels high in our bodies and the longer it stays at high levels, the more damage it can do to us.

Of all the hormones, cortisol has the most potential to damage our health. Furthermore, high cortisol has been found to be an influence in high blood pressure and Type II Diabetes, also called adult onset diabetes.[16] It is also implicated in the number one killer of women—heart disease. In an article by *Time* Magazine online, it was cited that, "heart disease is now the number one killer of women, striking every 1 in 3."[17] Killing one thousand four hundred women per day—half a million every year. More women under age forty-five die of heart disease than of any other disease. Among the causes listed are obesity, smoking, and stress.[18]

Despite our scientific achievements in society, it appears we have not caught up with ourselves physiologically in dealing with stress. We feel the pressures of our urban jungle environment and usually begin the "fight or flight" process.[19] People can experience stress and not even realize it. As I mentioned before, stress affects many bodily systems including the brain, hormones, organs and immune system.[20] The adrenal glands produce several hormones, including adrenaline and cortisol. Adrenaline gives us the push that we need to respond to stress, and cortisol modifies how our body uses fuel sources while under stress.[21] We actually need some cortisol to help us manage stress.

When we experience stress, cortisol stimulates protein to energy conversion, suppresses inflammation, and temporarily shuts down the immune system so that our body can handle the stress. After the stressful period, cortisol levels should go down and return to normal. However, if the stress does not go down, neither does the cortisol. It is this sustained high level of cortisol that is so damaging to our health.[22] Researchers have discovered correlations between elevated cortisol levels and increases in food cravings, body fat (specifically abdominal fat), and blood sugar levels. There also seems to be a relationship between elevated cortisol levels and reduced energy and sex drive, high blood pressure, memory problems, depression, anxiety disorders, decreased bone density and muscle mass, and disorders of premenstrual and menopausal symptoms.[23]

There are literally hundreds of books and publications about stress. When it came to cortisol, however, there was very little mainstream information. Once I was familiar with the term, I found a book written by Dr. Shawn Talbott called, *The Cortisol Connection: why stress makes you fat and ruins your health-and what you can do about it.* Wow! What a title—this summed it all up for me! This book defines the pathology of stress in the body. I would highly recommend this book to anyone who is experiencing prolonged stress or symptoms of chronic stress and would like to know how it can actually affect your health. Dr. Talbott wrote the book in a very factual and easy-to-understand style. By reading the book, I came to understand what cortisol really is and what it should and should not do.

Dr. Talbott describes both the typically stressed and chronically stressed lifestyles. I could definitely relate to the chronically stressed lifestyle. After reading his book, I was inspired to consult him, so I wrote to him. First I asked him why stress is so commonly diagnosed as depression. I wanted to know why so many doctors suggested I was depressed. I was well aware by now that stress could lead to depression. Had I not decided to explore the workings of chronic stress, I see how I could have developed depression from my symptoms. Doctor Talbott explained:

> Depression is often the initial diagnosis because it is a "quick fix" for doctors to treat stress. There are many drugs to treat depression, but no specific drugs are available to treat stress. Stress is not an illness, but rather a precursor to illness, and varies according to the person. There are many stressed out people with symptoms that are being treated inappropriately with antidepressants. Many people experience depression as a result of stress and high cortisol. Perhaps as much as 50 percent of depression is due to cortisol overexposure and the other half could possibly be attributed to problems with the neurotransmitter in the brain—serotonin. Existing antidepressant drugs work by increasing serotonin levels in the brain. The solution is not to mask the problem with drugs that increase serotonin, but rather to deal with the high cortisol and the reasons for the high stress—to go to the root of the problem.[24]

Humans are not equipped to deal with prolonged stress, but rather to deal with stress quickly and then return to a normal state.[25] Cortisol's role in the body is to maintain proper physiological processes while we are under stress to effectively deal with it. Hence, we cannot live without it.[26] If that was the case, I began to wonder—had high cortisol played a significant role in my health throughout my life, even as a child?

DO KIDS HAVE STRESS?

Children are not exempt from stress, but we often do not consider their stressors as significant as our adult stressors. In the book *The Ties That Stress—The New Family Imbalance*, author David Elkind concludes that, "most early studies of stress concentrated exclusively on adults." As a result he states: "stress was—and unfortunately to a large extent still is—regarded as a syndrome limited to adults."[27] Cortisol is present in our body throughout our whole lives—even as infants.

I read a brief article in Dr. James Dobson's *Focus on the Family* that described a study of a Harvard Medical School researcher, Dr. Mary Carlson. Dr. Carlson observed children and infants in a Romanian orphanage who lay in neglect due to overcrowding and an overworked staff. The children were hardly ever touched and lacked the nurturing they needed. What Dr. Carlson found especially alarming was that the children lay in the nursery in silence, without a cry or a sound. Her examination of the children who were about two years old revealed abnormally high levels of cortisol in their blood. High cortisol is known to cause brain damage, stunted growth, and developmental problems in children.[28]

I began to think cortisol could have played a role in my problem with sleep disturbances and night terrors as a child and with candida as a young teenager. With this information, it was now apparent that I could have been dealing with high cortisol ever since I was quite young. Research concludes that early life experiences are believed to lay the foundations of our stress response as we grow older, acting particularly on the systems in the body that react to stress, including the brain and nervous system. [29]

MASKING THE PROBLEM

In terms of the physiological response to stress, as I said before, both chronic stress and acute stress (fight or flight) can be damaging. Consider the effects of chronic stress to be more of a slow burn. Since individuals respond to stress differently, it is hard to measure stress. Damage caused by stress cannot be measured with any certainty; therefore, it continues to challenge medical researchers.

Two factors influence our ability to handle stress more than any others do: 1) the way we perceive the stressful event and 2) how healthy we are in order to manage the stress. The state of our physical health largely influences our ability to respond physiologically to stress.[30]

When was the last time you asked yourself how you're feeling? I asked myself this question all the time. I did not smoke, drank only on rare social occasions, exercised, and even watched what I ate; nevertheless, I was suffering from symptoms with origins most doctors could not explain, so I was forced to find them out myself. I wondered how many others followed in my footsteps, running back and forth to doctors who would treat symptoms of something much more complex than they had realized. In virtually no time, you find yourself taking medication for every single symptom, without doctors putting much effort into investigating the root of the problem. Because stress can lead to depression, I could understand why doctors "fix" the problems of stress with psychotropic drugs. Taking antidepressants made me feel more relaxed—they somewhat numbed the symptoms, but if I stopped taking them, my symptoms still existed. It was only a band-aid solution; it was not a cure.

Antidepressants work by increasing the hormone serotonin in the brain. Stress decreases serotonin levels in the brain.[31] Serotonin is the hormone that makes us feel good, relaxed, calm, and satisfied. Upon researching, I found statistics for the use of antidepressants to be alarming! In an article published in the *Annals of Pharmacotherapy*, the authors reported that the use of prescription antidepressants had increased 353 percent from 1981 to 2000 in Canada.[32] No, that's not a typo—you read correctly—a 353 percent increase! Some experts believe that over one million Canadians are clinically depressed and that one in four women are taking prescription antidepressants. Studies suggest that we should be concerned about these drugs because they have shown that some of the most commonly prescribed antidepressants (Elavil and Prozac) promote mammary tumor growth—cancer—in laboratory studies. Studies have also shown that another popular antidepressant (Paxil) caused a seven-fold increase in the risk of breast cancer.[33] According to some estimates, the use of psychotropic drugs (stimulants, sleeping pills, relaxants) in the United States alone almost rivals that of the entire world combined.[34] The question is: are we depressed or are we chronically stressed? What's the difference?

CHRONIC STRESS VS. DEPRESSION

Having a cold, the flu, or malaria can all produce some of the same symptoms, but clearly, they are different illnesses in their severity and complexity of symptoms, as well as their outcomes. While people have died from all three, most can withstand the common cold. The flu presents more challenging symptoms with greater severity, and malaria, even more. The same could then be said for chronic stress and depression. Both can produce similar symptoms, yet chronic stress is not depression.

It is my opinion that chronic stress is being over-looked and misdiagnosed as depression simply because fixing chronic stress requires an entire lifestyle change with much more commitment from both the doctor and patient. On the other hand, patients more readily accept depression diagnoses because they provide for quick relief by using drugs. So, is there a big difference between depression and chronic stress?

With this question, I went to the pros at the Toronto-based Canadian Institute of Stress, founded in 1979 in part by stress pioneer, Dr. Hans Selye. I asked Director Dr. Richard Earle what the difference was between chronic stress and depression. He explained that, "because chronic stress and depression have the same biological basis, they are often diagnosed as the same." This, however, does not imply that they are the same. Dr. Earle elaborated, "Whereas depression is a clinical diagnosis, [chronic] stress is simply a bio-psychological human condition...not a legitimate diagnosis." [35]

The accepted medical definition of clinical depression lists specific requirements for its diagnosis. In her book *Outsmarting Female Fatigue: 8 Strategies for Lifelong Vitality*, author Debra Waterhouse describes five "tell-tale signs of depression." She lists: "1) difficulty doing the things you've always done, 2) hopeless feelings about the future, 3) difficulty when making decisions, 4) a feeling of worthlessness, and 5) not enjoying the things you used to enjoy."[36] When considering these key indicators of depression, my symptoms did not match these signs.

Though I was discouraged and run down, I never felt hopeless or worthless; I was able to do the things I had always done, granted I was extremely exhausted, and I did not experience any difficulty making decisions. The author goes on to state that "brief periods of sadness, indecision or hopelessness are normal, but just because you have these five characteristics of depression doesn't mean you need anti-depressants or therapy at this point, it may only mean you just need something pleasurable to balance your emotional state."[37] True depression is a definable, clinical illness characterized by at a minimum the five key signs listed above and sometimes by a host of other symptoms as well, including decreased sex drive, lethargy, difficulty concentrating, and even digestive problems.[38]

Although severe stress can bring on depression, it is only one of its many causes. Another definition of depression I found was clearly not what I had been experiencing: "depression is a severe state of unhappiness that imposes itself on a person's state of mind and affects his or her habits and normal conduct for at least two consecutive weeks."[39] I did not feel this serious unhappiness, nor was I experiencing any change in my habits, especially at work. Work allowed for little rest; I had to keep going. Although I was overworked, discouraged, and even sad at times, I had always held on to one thought in my mind—hope! Maybe hope was the footprint in the sands of my life thus far—maybe someone else had been carrying me.

DID CORTISOL MAKE ME DO IT?

One day, I was having a particularly stressful morning at work, and when I left my desk for lunch, I headed straight for the candy aisle! This day, (I laugh about it now because I actually caught myself) I felt like a healthy snack was just not going to cut it. I needed sugar! I wanted something sweet to cure my mood. I left the store with a bag of chocolate-covered coconut bars and ate them all at once. I felt better for about ten minutes. Then, I sulked in guilt. I knew all this candy was no good for me. Then it dawned on me, I had had a stressful morning, and the first thing I went for was sugar. If it was not sugar, it would have been something fatty, greasy, or otherwise unhealthy treat because that is what I felt like eating. I felt bad, so I wanted something good tasting, but not good for me.

This reminded me of the time my sister called from her cell phone sounding very upset. I was concerned at first but then laughed in the end. She was having one of those days and admitted (like in a confessional) that she had driven straight to Burger King, ordered a chicken sandwich, and ate the whole thing! In our family, Burger King chicken sandwiches are reserved for extreme cases of stress or for a very special occasion. Here she was, bawling on the phone, saying she had one nerve left, and she drove it to Burger King!

I had to laugh; I really did. Not because she was having a bad day, but because she was more upset about having inhaled a chicken sandwich than she was about whatever had stressed her out in the first place. I assured her it was fine considering her stressful circumstances (as though I was the judge of the case) and that she should calm down and relax. Ironic! Here I was telling someone to calm down and relax, when I was the one on the big journey toward understanding stress! However, I did notice people's tendency under stress, including myself, to head straight for the junk food.

I came across this very subject while reading more about cortisol. I found many articles and papers in journals that described very technical tests and analyses of cortisol. Much of the scientific evidence showed high cortisol producing adverse effects on human health. I was specifically interested in articles that related cortisol to eating patterns and obesity. One article discussed a study of healthy women exposed to laboratory stressors. The women who experienced greater stress levels in the test subsequently ate more. Thus, the results suggested that women who were more vulnerable to stress could potentially be at risk for weight gain due to cortisol reactivity.[40] I wondered if this could be the reason I had been gaining weight, why I succumbed to the chocolate coconut bars, or, like my sister, the drive-thru window for the "forbidden" chicken sandwich. Could stress be making me feel hungry and prompting me to eat more? How did it actually do this in my body? Could there be some strange chemical process subconsciously driving me to a snack attack?

FEEDING STRESS!

I urge you to take a look around you the next time you are, say, in a shopping mall or a restaurant. Without being judgmental, you will not have to look far before noticing how many people are overweight. Obesity is on the rise and getting worse. Studies suggest that elevated cortisol may be contributing to the phenomenon of "stress-eating."[41] Researchers now consider obesity to be an epidemic, particularly in Western society and parts of Europe.[42] Obesity is not socially acceptable, and most people consider it a problem of willpower, rather than an actual disease. However, more recent studies suggest that obesity could be a disease of energy regulation, the notion that we are taking in more energy than we are using.

Insulin resistance is also associated with obesity and physical inactivity.[43] The body's cells need insulin to absorb glucose. If this absorption is not working properly, the body increases insulin secretion and causes fluctuating blood sugar levels. If this condition goes untreated, it can develop into Type II diabetes or other diseases.[44] Other researchers have noted that high cortisol linked to insulin resistance is often present in cases of abdominal obesity.[45] I noticed this in my mirror, though I was not overweight by any standard. Still, I looked like I had a life preserver of fat around my middle! Studies now suggest a correlation between cortisol exposure (that is, too much cortisol secretion) and increased food intake.[46]

Even die-hard dieters with high-stress lifestyles cannot seem to shake the excess flab! Why? Because stress and the subsequent high release of stress hormones, including cortisol, seem to encourage fat retention in the body, even if you diet and exercise religiously. Stress invokes a response in our bodies similar to that of starvation; the body feels the stress, so it begins to conserve energy by storing more calories as fat.

As if that were not bad enough, stress also changes where the body stores fat. Hence, many people who diet and exercise, but have high stress, still seem to store fat in the abdominal region, rather than the legs or hips, which is particularly true for women.[47] Middle fat, (the fat in the stomach area) also called visceral fat, is structurally different from the fat in other areas of the body. More blood flows in the fatty area of the middle, and there are more glucocorticoid (stress hormone) receptors in this area. As cortisol flows through this fatty area, it increases in size.[48] The more stress we feel, the more cortisol we produce; the more cortisol we produce, the more fat we store!

So, the vicious cycle begins. We diet and exercise more, paying more attention to these two areas, rather than to the chronic high stress we are experiencing every day. Moreover, when we do not get the results we expect, we often diet more and exercise harder, only exacerbating the stress and gaining more weight. It is frustrating and downright discouraging. We often do not see the real reason for the weight retention (chronic stress) because we are so focused on the results of our frantic diet and exercise regime. If, however, we considered toning down the underlying stress, we would find we could begin to achieve the results that diet and exercise alone could not bring.

In North America, obesity is at an all-time high. Besides the obvious problem of high levels of refined sugar and simple carbohydrates in the Western diet, stress could be the next consideration in the problem of obesity. However, health experts say very little about the stress connection. They constantly blame us for what and how much we eat, yet, unless we are searching for the deeper reasons, we will not hear much about how stress relates to eating.

There is no doubt that poor diets are a factor in the decline of our health.[49] Fast food and convenience foods are the major culprits for Americans, who spent more than one hundred ten billion dollars on fast food in the year 2000.[50] The average North American consumes approximately one hundred fifty pounds of sugar a year![51] In stark contrast, Americans are spending close to forty billion dollars per year on dieting and weight loss procedures, plus a staggering seventy billion dollars a year in weight-related healthcare costs.[52] A report issued by the World Health Organization states: "There are more than one billion adults worldwide who are overweight and at least three hundred million who are clinically obese. Among these, about half a million people in North America and Western Europe combined will die from obesity-related diseases."[53] Statistics Canada released in 2003 show that 14.9 percent of Canadians are obese and 33.3 percent are overweight, with a total healthcare cost of over 1.8 billion dollars.[54]

Emotional issues are directly involved in what we eat. Furthermore, if we eat and how we eat strongly relates to stress.[55] Now researchers are even finding a connection between what we eat and increased cortisol levels. Recent studies reveal drinking two or three cups of coffee per day can increase cortisol levels.[56] Cortisol levels increase after we eat because food stimulates the HPA axis.[57] The HPA axis, as previously mentioned, is the hypothalamic-pituitary-adrenal system of endocrine glands that intercede in the response to stress.[58] Abnormalities of this system have direct effects on insulin resistance and weight gain.[59] High cortisol levels in the body are "*extremely corrosive,*" especially to heart tissue and the hypothalamus area of the brain.[60] Could this be why heart disease is the number one killer of women or why diagnoses of depression and mental illnesses have skyrocketed?

Although much more research needs to be done on the phenomenon of "stress-eating," substantial scientific evidence suggests that increased stress and increased stress hormones, specifically cortisol, play a significant role in our eating habits. Stereotypically, women are often targeted as stress-eaters. See for yourself. The next time you watch a favorite sitcom or movie with a female protagonist, perhaps after a romantic break-up or the loss of a great job opportunity, you'll see her indulging in comfort food (typically ice cream—a whole pint of it!) while tears are flowing or angry words are flying. The scene quickly changes from the cause of the stress to the girl, the ice cream, and her spoon!

We have learned to associate our stress with eating. Advertisers know what we want and have created fun names for flavors and treats to entice the "emotional" appetite of nibblers. When we are sad, we gravitate to "feel good" foods like ice cream or chocolate. When we feel angry, we often crunch on some snack foods to release the anger and aggression. No doubt, food can be a comfort we enjoy, but it seems the more stress we have, the more comfort we need and the more food it takes to fulfill it. We are not eating simply because of hunger or nutritional needs, but for many other reasons. While we are all likely guilty of the "bad day" binge, statistics on obesity and weight-related illnesses tell us a different story. It seems there are just too many "bad days."

THE IMMUNE SYSTEM

The immune system is "one of the surveillance systems of the body." The purpose of the immune system is to detect and rid the body of potential infection. It is in constant motion, detecting and protecting the body against anything that should not be there. Without an immune system, we could not live.[61] We should think of our immune system as a guard at the gate of our health.

If you have ever experienced stress, then you have also felt the effects of stress hormones, including cortisol. When we experience stress, our blood pressure rises, our heart beat increases, and our muscles get tense. All of our senses activate under stress.[62] However, when we are experiencing stress, we do not often think of our immune system protecting us. We are mostly preoccupied with treating symptoms while we ignore the underlying factors. The immune system provides protection and defense against disease. There are many parts to the immune system which all must be working together to maintain proper balance for it to function. If one or more parts are impaired or not functioning properly, then the immune system is "compromised," allowing disease to enter.[63]

The components of the immune system are rather detailed and complex; however, it is worth mentioning that the immune system operates hand-in-hand with other bodily systems. These include the central nervous system and the autonomic nervous system (being the sympathetic and parasympathetic nervous systems).[64] Concerning stress, exposure to a stress stimulus, whether it is emotional or physical (such as an infection) initiates a complex series of responses in the body designed to protect and restore stability. Scientists and medical professionals call this stability homeostasis. Laypersons and others refer to it as balance. The HPA axis plays a very important role in maintaining homeostasis (balance). When the HPA axis is not functioning properly, a host of disorders can result, affecting physical and mental function. It can affect growth, metabolism, and reproductive ability, as well as the ability to cope effectively with stress.[65]

Failure to respond properly to stress can be quite dangerous and can be a significant contributing factor to diseases such as cardiovascular disorders, gastrointestinal difficulties, and psychological conditions, as well as to complications in immune function.[66] Glucocorticoids (anti-inflammatory hormones like cortisol) have the ability to change the functions of all cells within the immune system, potentially resulting in a suppressed immune system.[67]

Today, there is more increased interest in research about the relationship of stress to the immune system. This is mostly because of the multidisciplinary approach, in which scientists study the immune system along with the endocrine, psychological, behavioral, and autonomic systems. Cortisol has become the most studied of the stress hormones that affect the immune system. Yet, it is a hormone that most people have never even heard of.[68] Nevertheless, in our stress-saturated culture, we had better start to understand more about this and other stress hormones and their effects—particularly on women.

CORTISOL AND SLEEP

I started to suspect cortisol was a factor in my sleep disturbances. After having my cortisol levels check, I contacted the doctors that had performed my latest sleep test. I told them I had found out that my cortisol levels were high and wondered if this was related to my sleep problems. They indicated that high cortisol could definitely be a factor in my sleeping pattern since cortisol was supposed to increase as we wake in the morning. Gradually it should lower throughout the day and into the night, allowing us to sleep. In my case, cortisol levels were high in the morning and remained high throughout the day. This meant it was quite possible the levels were still high during the night, when I should be asleep.

I knew that cortisol was not likely the sole factor in the symptoms I was experiencing, but I was convinced, as were my doctors, that it was playing a leading role in my health problems. I was able to correlate most of my symptoms to high stress levels, but I was still puzzled as to how candida fit in.

6

Controversial Candida

Nothing I had researched before would be as revealing as candida syndrome. The condition of candida is still one of the most controversial medical subjects in modern medicine. Some doctors are completely convinced it exists, while others argue that it does not. There is much conflicting medical opinion about it. Doctors sometimes refer to Candida syndrome as dysbiosis (flora imbalance). It is most commonly known as yeast overgrowth. It is caused by an imbalance of bacteria in the body. Bacteria naturally occur in the body and are found in our skin, nails, mouth, gut, and mucous membranes.

While researching about problems with sleep and headaches, I stumbled across candida by accident. I had battled this problem for many years. However, it never occurred to me to think it could be contributing to my long-term symptoms.

While searching for information about stress hormones, I came across the website of Dr. Michael Biamonte in New York. Dr. Biamonte describes many symptoms and correlates them to candidiasis (yeast overgrowth). The list of symptoms and problems associated with *Candida* overgrowth was startling. I decided to take a closer look at candida syndrome.

As authors and doctors in the treatment of chronic candidiasis, John Parks Trowbridge and Morton Walker were all too familiar with the difficulty of diagnosing this confusing condition. In their book *The Yeast Syndrome*, they conclude:

> Patients with complex and often conflicting symptoms may end up seeing [many different doctors and specialists] seeking relief for the symptoms of the yeast syndrome, but because their symptoms are not specific to any disease state, they are often passed on to another doctor or convinced that their symptoms are all in their head.[1]

This was me! That is exactly how I felt for years. I could relate to the frustration of bouncing from doctor to doctor, not being clinically sick, yet not feeling well either. Again, I had no idea that an overgrowth of yeast could potentially produce and exacerbate my symptoms. It had never occurred to me that yeast overgrowth, itself, was part of the problem. Add to this that it is not easy to recognize candida.

Much controversy surrounds the idea that *Candida* is related to a pool of illnesses and symptoms, including acne, allergies, anxiety, constipation, depression, premenstrual syndrome (PMS), headaches, fatigue, joint pain, muscle weakness, persistent cough, rashes and other skin irritations, insomnia, vaginitis, memory problems, infertility and lost sex drive.[2] This is not the complete list, but it was enough to prompt me to continue researching. The difficulty in diagnosing candida with these symptoms is that these very symptoms may occur in other areas of disease and illness. If you are not specifically looking for it, it can go undetected, and even worse, misdiagnosed. Not surprisingly, no doctor I saw ever suggested this irritating disease could potentially be very serious. I was consistently given prescriptions to treat localized infections, and consistently, I returned with the same problem for years. It was not until I understood the condition of candida that I was able to correlate it to my own health.

Most women feel embarrassed discussing or admitting they have trouble with candida; however, considering that reports indicate that over twenty-two million American women suffer from this problem recurringly[3], women need desperately to address this problem. Candida can produce a variety of symptoms. If you have ever dealt with this menace, then you know how irritating and stubborn it can be. It often leaves you feeling there is no relief in sight. Originally, researchers thought it was primarily a problem for women; however, more modern research shows that men and children are just as susceptible to yeast overgrowth as women.[4] Thus, understanding this bacterial imbalance is the first step in knowing how to get rid of it!

To eliminate any confusion, I should explain that we all have fungi and bacteria in our bodies. Like cortisol, we are supposed to have some. Yeast is a one-celled organism capable of reproducing asexually by budding. Just *one* yeast organism is capable of reproducing into billions. Yeast thrives in warm, dark, moist environments and cluster together in the body.[5] Candida syndrome and specifically the yeast called *Candida albicans* have the ability to cause symptoms within nine different systems of the body (the endocrine, musculoskeletal, nervous, digestive, lymphatic, respiratory, urinary, cardiovascular and reproductive systems).[6] Normally present in the body, yeast is controlled by our immune system and by "friendly" bacteria. If changes occur that disrupt the balance of these bacteria, then the immune system becomes compromised, and the "friendly" bacteria decrease. This allows the yeast organisms to grow rapidly, take over, and wreak havoc.[7]

Yeast thrives on fats and sugars, two staples of the typical Western diet.[8] As if that were not enough, yeast is very sneaky. Over time, it is able to change from the yeast phase to a fungal phase that releases toxins in the body. In the fungal form, yeast burrow into the mucous membranes, specifically the intestinal tract. The yeast can now become systemic (entering the bloodstream)[9] growing rapidly in the body, spreading like wildfire to virtually any organ or tissue.[10] Fungi feed off dead and diseased tissue; therefore, a yeast or fungal infection is usually a sign of immune suppression and jeopardized health.[11] With the widespread use of antibiotics, anti-inflammatory drugs, and birth control pills, North Americans are particularly afflicted with fungal infections which are rising annually at epidemic proportions.[12] Cortisone also greatly increases the growth of fungi in the body.[13] This, I found to be particularly interesting. Was there a connection between cortisol and candida syndrome?

CORTISOL AND *CANDIDA*

Yeast overgrowth is not a new problem. It has been around for ages. What I found interesting is that yeast overgrowth can profoundly invade the body's tissues. It can also extensively damage the organs. Yeast is an extremely aggressive organism.[14] It's unique resilience became famous during the 1940's and 1950's when yeast organisms had apparently survived the fallout of nuclear bomb testing![15]

Yeast has the amazing capability of building molecules that mimic hormonal molecules. Yeast is very clever! It can enter our body's cellular system, interrupt the metabolic processes within and ravage our health.[16] Yeast creates antigens in the body. Antigens are substances that stimulate the production of antibodies. These antigens work against our natural enzymes and hormones, which are normally beneficial.[17] Also, as yeast grow, they multiply by the millions and billions, releasing toxins as they thrive. These toxins have a direct, negative effect on the endocrine (hormonal) system, the nervous system, and especially, the immune system.[18] *Candida* overgrowth can be quite severe because it produces these toxins when the body is already compromised by other factors that can weaken the immune system, such as nutritional deficiencies, environmental pollutants and stress.[19]

When we are under stress, high levels of stress hormones, including cortisol, are pumping through the body, causing serotonin levels to decrease. When serotonin levels decrease, we do not feel as good or energetic as we normally would, and sometimes we even feel melancholy or sad. It is then that we often crave sweet foods and carbohydrates for quick energy and quick mood fixes. It is the resulting dietary effects of our stress-induced eating that can exacerbate candida symptoms. We feed the stress with the very things that yeast thrive on...sugar, fat, and simple carbohydrates.

"You Have to Seek It Out"

With physicians so divided on the topic of candida, it is hard to get the advice you need. On one hand, some doctors are very "candida-concerned," while others dismiss the claims that it can wreak havoc on our health. I wanted to know why candida was often misdiagnosed and why many doctors are skeptical about it. I contacted Dr. Michael Biamonte at his clinic, The Biamonte Center for Clinical Nutrition, in Manhattan. Dr. Biamonte is a certified clinical nutritionist. He has treated hundreds of patients with candida, as well as chronic fatigue syndrome, viruses, and other infectious illnesses. He explained that, "the testing for *Candida* is relatively new and generally not done by the conventional labs that most MD's use. Mostly labs that cater to naturopathic doctors, alternative medicine specialists, etcetera, do it. One would need to seek it out!"

I also asked him why many doctors were skeptical about the possibility of *Candida* being a contributor to many health problems. He replied:

> There are two theories: first, why would they want to admit to the existence of an illness if they (themselves) are causing by prescribing antibiotics and hormones. Second, the data on candidiasis and its symptoms has not been "headlined" in the Journal of the American

Medical Association, the nations' mouthpiece for MD's. However, the data does exist if you search it out!

Dr. Biamonte believes that, "as much as 30 percent of the population of the United States alone will experience candidiasis," and indicates that, "some patients will overcome it on their own and others would have to seek professional help."[20]

Self-education is the key. Learning about diet, nutrition, and exercise, as well as vitamin and mineral supplements and stress relief and relaxation techniques are essential to maintaining quality health. In my case, I took the advice of Dr. Biamonte and my naturopath and followed their instruction. With a proper diet and essential vitamin and mineral supplements my health improved. I soon became aware of the "triggers" to avoid in combating this condition and learned how to eliminate it from my system. Soon, I had fewer symptoms of yeast overgrowth; moreover, I had increased health and vitality. I had more energy, fewer headaches, and less fatigue. I began to lose weight and experience deeper and more relaxed sleep. This was something I had not felt in years. It was hard to believe how long I had suffered with these recurring symptoms. Yet, once I understood the nature of my problem and took the time to educate myself, I was able to begin reversing my condition. I had not invested this kind of time in anything other than work. Now, I was taking as much time as necessary to correct my health problems. It was really beginning to pay off!

COULD CANDIDA BE YOUR PROBLEM?

Many people might be reading this and thinking, "I've never had trouble with bacterial imbalance." Yet, studies show that almost 75 percent of women alone will experience at least one episode of candida in their lifetime, with many developing recurring problems afterwards.[21]

Numerous studies also indicate that yeast overgrowth and gastrointestinal bacterial imbalances have been responsible for, or at least exaggerated, the conditions of many illnesses. Some researchers have found connections between candidiasis and Crohn's, colitis, irritable bowel syndrome, diabetes, lupus, multiple sclerosis, fibromyalgia and chronic fatigue syndrome, as well as children's disorders such as attention deficit disorder and attention deficit hyperactive disorder. With this list, it becomes more difficult for people to deny that bacterial imbalances are not a contributing factor to ill health. The most dangerous and significant aspect of this condition is it's ability to escape the intestinal tract and become blood borne—potentially invading many other parts of the body.[22] Once this happens, it can seriously affect your health—as it had for years with me. Over forty million Americans have systemic fungal infections, so yeast and bacterial overgrowth play a larger role in our health than most people realize. We usually treat infections with antibiotics, but antibiotics create conditions in which yeast and other fungi flourish, adding fuel to the fire. Because yeast is a normal part of the humans' gastrointestinal tracts, yeast overgrowth and bacterial imbalances can affect both males and females of any age.[23]

Diagnostic laboratories and alternative practitioners are now putting more effort into developing specific tests for *Candida* overgrowth and dysbiosis. Tests to determine *Candida* growth counts, as well as many new treatment options are now available. If you suspect you could be suffering from candida, it is best to look for a specialist who will address your concerns and determine specific testing procedures and proper diagnosis. Candida is curable and practitioners who understand the dietary and lifestyle changes needed to combat this frustrating condition are readily available for those who are determined to find relief.

CANDIDA AND CHRONIC FATIGUE SYNDROME

Fatigue is a common complaint among many patients, particularly women. In writing this book, I became more interested in how many people were concerned about feeling tired all the time. Studies have shown that both chronic candida syndrome (CCS) and chronic fatigue syndrome (CFS) also called chronic fatigue immune dysfunction syndrome (CFIDS) have many of the same symptoms, but unlike CFS, candidiasis does not always produce the sudden flu-like symptoms typically associated with chronic fatigue. Both conditions seem to lead to the same immunological result since both suppress immune function. One study suggested "chronic candidiasis of the intestine and other mucosal sites may be a causal factor for immune dysfunction in a significant percentage of patients with CFS, and in some cases a necessary precursor for CFS."[24]

With this knowledge, I could identify a pattern in myself. I made the connection between fatigue due to high stress and cortisol and yeast overgrowth. *Candida* and cortisol were living a sordid relationship in my body for years! My immune system had become so weak it was no match against *Candida*. To my surprise, I read medical studies that made a direct connection between chronic candida and chronic fatigue-immune deficiency. Again, not one doctor ever mentioned this connection to me. Not once did they suggest that the symptoms of candida I had experienced might indicate that my immune system was worn down.

I simply got used to feeling run down. Had I known chronic stress and high stress hormones had contributed so much to my experiencing fatigue, headaches, hypoglycemia, insomnia, and finally—candida, I would have made the effort much earlier in life to rectify the problem. I had now found a strong link to each of my symptoms.

7

What Is Stressing Us?

I took this question back to my research group of women. I received many responses, but the most predominant response was that women generally felt deprived of time. They did not have enough time to get everything done. They did not have time to exercise, to eat better, and to spend time with their children, spouses, and partners. They had no time to for themselves. On top of all that, these women were tired—very, very tired—exhausted, in fact. Of the many possible stressors, time and money had the greatest influence. In this chapter, I share the feedback of these women, which covers some of the greatest causes of chronic stress for women today.

PRISONERS OF TIME

I've been on a calendar—but I've never been on time.
—Marilyn Monroe

You cannot stop it, hang on to it, slow it down, or make it disappear. This commodity that we spend too quickly and try so hard to save is none other than time. We are a society out of time, running late, and needing it yesterday! It seems the one thing we want more of, other than money, is time. We may even want as much time now, as we do money (as I concluded from my mini-survey in Chapter 4). How is it we have advanced technologically, but regressed in the use of our time?

The old promises of technology to allow us unlimited free time, are still, empty promises. We were led to believe the myth that as machines replaced more and more labor, we would have much more free time. Although many machines have replaced the need for people, we seem to be busier now than ever before.

So, what are we doing with all our time? In his book, *Ritalin Nation*, Dr. Richard DeGrandpre devotes the entire first chapter to what he describes as, "[t]he hurried society." Dr. DeGrandpre blames the rise in big technological advances throughout the past few decades for the hyperactive, sensationalized, and over-stimulated population that we are today. He specifically calls this "rapid-fire culture…a nation strung out on excitement…where leisure, slowness, idleness, relaxation and simplicity have all become pastimes of American (Western) culture."[1] I could relate. He describes time as no longer being something we enjoy, but rather a thing which stands between us and what we would like to be doing or what we envision for our lives. Time feels more like "an obstacle in our pursuit of happiness."[2]

Time was something I just never seemed to have—or, was I was not paying attention to it? With the ever-diminishing quantity and quality of time, the foundation of our families, marriages, and relationships are falling apart. Often because we are usually in a hurry or because we are not satisfied with what we have, we always seem to want more. Because we want more "stuff" and have increased social demands, we have more work and less free time. With the desire and need for more, many couples feel they need two incomes, so in many families, both parents work. This has caused a huge strain on family dynamics, as well as a reduction in the quality of life for women.

Women are often stretched beyond their limits in order to achieve their own goals or to provide the necessary comforts for their families. How do we do it all? And, what about all the stress this can cause? Dr.

DeGrandpre suggests that "a higher standard of living sets the stage for a better quality of life, perhaps, but it does not guarantee one." He goes on to say that, "despite the fact that America is considered the most powerful and advanced nation in the world, we have yet to investigate seriously the factors contributing to mental health and personal contentment."[3]

"Just Take a Pill!"

> *Medicine is a collection of uncertain prescriptions the results of which, taken collectively, are more fatal than useful to mankind.*
>
> —Napoleon

There was a saying amongst teenagers during my years in high school that would be wonderful if it were possible: "Take a stress-tab." This would be a perfect solution to our modern, hectic, stress-soaked lifestyles. If only there were a pill, a one-dose method of reducing or relieving stress—it would be the top-selling prescription, and the creator would be one lucky billionaire! Unfortunately, for most, stress does not go away with the popping of one pill. Instead, it is muted in a "cocktail" of prescriptions that relieve pain, reduce inflammation, increase energy, improve sleep, and assist with psychological functioning. Enter painkillers, anti-inflammatories, stimulants (uppers), tranquilizers (downers), sleeping pills, muscle relaxants, antidepressants—you name it!

It takes several medications to treat the symptoms of stress because stress is multifaceted. The "just take a pill" mentality has become a daily way of life for many. Medicines and prescriptions, however, are not always the answer, especially when dealing with the effects of chronic stress. Compare stress to an onion; you must peel back the layers to get to the root. You have to go through each symptom layer and identify its origin. Because stress manifests itself in so many different ways, it requires a tenacious approach to understanding how to reduce it and regain control of your life.

WE LOSE CONTROL

Control is a word fraught with emotional connotations. To lose control indicates instability, with instability comes fear of the unknown. We are not a society that copes well with powerlessness or instability. As babies, we learn that our actions can significantly control circumstances around us. When we cry, someone feeds us. As toddlers, we throw tantrums and often get our way because our parents want to avoid the embarrassing scene we are causing in the grocery aisle. Then, as teenagers, we attempt to control our parents with our demands or silent withdrawal and we seek control again amongst our peers by conforming and trying to "fit in." While we control ourselves through learning and instinct, if we take on more than we can handle, things get out of control.

This lack of control allows stress to enter and begins undermining the stability we work so hard to establish. Then, instability begets fear. Here, I am reminded of a psychology course I took in college. While I yawned through Freud's theories, I sat up intrigued by those of Abraham Maslow with his "Hierarchy of Needs" (and I thought I'd never use that information again!). Maslow claimed that humans had five general needs, which he presented in the form of a pyramid. The most important or essential needs were at the base, and the most complete and ideal were at the top. His hierarchy begins with physiological (basic needs of food, water, air, sleep, and sex), moves on to safety, love, and esteem (competence and recognition) and peaks with self-actualization (a desire to do and become more). According to Maslow, stability and safety are second only to physiological needs.

He concluded that we all strive to satisfy these needs and that if we cannot satisfy them, we become sick. He explains that we must meet the lower needs (basic needs) before we are motivated to satisfy the higher needs (like self esteem).[4] This is apparent when you look at impoverished and underprivileged societies where basic needs are lacking. These people lack a sense of security, which in turn lowers their self-esteem and results in further disadvantages and discord.

How does this relate to stress? Stress causes worry, anxiety, and weariness, and vice versa. Because we are not satisfied, we do not feel secure. Whatever is stressing us makes us feel that we are lacking something we need. It may be that we have too much work or are out of work, have too much responsibility or too little responsibility. Worse yet, we may not have time to satisfy our basic needs (as listed above) so that our higher needs suffer as well. If one level of the pyramid deteriorates, the whole thing starts to collapse. A good example is the stressed out woman! Women are frequently more susceptible to stress than men because of their desire to nurture, tend to others, care for children and homes, and maintain careers.

When women spend so much time taking care of the needs of others, they often neglect their own needs. Many women I spoke to about this said that they felt a large sense of guilt when they indulged in themselves instead of their children, spouses, and even extended family. A woman "treats" herself to what has become adopted as "luxuries" that are mostly just the basic needs of satisfaction according to Maslow, for instance a cup of tea, a walk for fresh air, or a quiet night alone with her spouse or partner. She often has to do without these so-called "basic" needs because of the demands and needs of so many around her. We see the domino effect occur in Maslow's pyramid: the woman's ability for self-actualization diminishes; she begins to lose self-esteem which can affect her love life (sheer exhaustion and lack of interest); hence, her relationships and companionships suffer and eventually, she becomes emotionally drained, physically exhausted, and psychologically distraught. Unfortunately, it seems the most common way to treat this is with a diagnosis of "depression" and the subsequent use of anti-depressant drugs.

SISTERS OF PERPETUAL MOTION

No, not the religious sisters found in a monastery or nunnery, but your friends, co-workers, mothers, sisters, and the women around you every day. In physics, the theory of perpetual motion is the concept that a machine will run forever, without breaking down, never requiring refueling, or recharging. Still, it is a theory considered impossible. The idea that something could continually operate without ever needing to re-energize is still the stuff of dreams in energy science. However, this idea is evident with the rising and setting of the sun, which is seemingly endless.[5]

Society often operates with the idea that we are beings of perpetual motion, especially women. We do not stop to realize that we cannot accomplish everything we "need" to do. Although we were designed to move, we were not designed to remain in motion! Physics should redefine the theory of perpetual motion to read: See women! We spend so much time taking care of others, that our basic needs take the back seat, even on good days. We feel the stress of it all, and become sick. This follows Maslow's theory and Hans Selye's conclusion that when the demands are too high, we break down.

I asked the same group of women I had researched with a new question. I asked what they wished they had more time for in life. I stated it as: "I wish I had more time for _____" and asked them to fill in the blank. I was interested to see how many responses correlated with what Maslow would describe as a basic need (air, water, food, sex, and sleep). I also included exercise in this category because I considered it a basic need for health and well being.

The responses were generally all the same: most women indicated they wanted more time for themselves. They wanted more time to take care of themselves, to enjoy the things that made them feel better, happier, and healthier. Popular responses included: more time with their spouses or partners (including sex—basic need), more time to exercise (basic need), and more time for things like friends and hobbies. I am not sure where Maslow might include friends or hobbies, but I am convinced that women need more of the basic needs of this hierarchy than ever before. Although the needs of these women seemed to vary, the one common response was that they all wanted (and needed) more time.

YOU'VE COME A LONG WAY BABY—(BUT…JUST KEEP GOING)!

Despite the fact that women have come a long way since the days when they burned their bras in an attempt to gain more independence, rights, and freedoms, we are still very much living in a man's world. Women today are under a great deal of pressure, and the health statistics support this picture—women are sick, women are dying, and women are developing more diseases like cancer, heart disease, and depression. Inequality, harassment, and discrimination still follow women like a shadow. Even medically, women often struggle to be considered more than a man with a uterus. Women's health should be clearly distinguished from men's health. If we are going to understand and develop preventative methods for the statistically high number of diseases that are afflicting women today, then we need to understand women's needs better.

I'm often interested in reading news clips or articles about women in the workforce. Many women, even those in positions of power, like managers, CEO's and political leaders, are often underpaid, under appreciated, or both, in comparison to their male counterparts. Those in power often subliminally punish or withhold civil rights from women. Whether it is maternity leave or issues of equality, you would think that with the way we have advanced as a society, we would have recognized women's equality better by now. However, women's inequalities seem to be just as present today as before; they are just not as obvious. Many women still encounter difficulties or negative attitudes in the workplace when they become pregnant, and perhaps even have to fight corporate politics and administration for weeks or even months! For this reason, some companies prefer to hire men rather than women.

Whichever choice women make, it seems eventually, someone will label them inappropriately. The expectation to be both a career woman and a mother and wife is often a burden. For those who choose the career path, the label can be rather harsh. Some people consider women selfish if they pursue a career instead of marriage and motherhood. On the other hand, many people consider housewives and stay-at-home moms either spoiled or non-productive and imagine them lounging around eating bon-bons and watching soap operas! Negative stereotypes about women seem to stick with them over time. Should we be surprised then to find that statistics reveal women are more predisposed to diagnoses of depression and anxiety disorders? Dr. David Sheehan, author of *The Anxiety Disease*, suggests, *"anxiety is more prevalent than depression, and eighty percent of those who suffer from it are women."*[6] Diseases like depression and schizophrenia, and a host of other disorders such as obsessive-compulsive disorder have increased more in the latter part of this century than at any time before.[7]

TOXIC PEOPLE!

Chances are, if I asked you to name one person described by each of the following categories, you could name several: demanding boss, snippy co-worker, obnoxious neighbor, or stereotypical mother-in-law. Toxic people are people who you dread interacting with. They are the people who make you want to scream, "You make me sick!" Only, we would not actually say that unless we were upset enough. However, you should evaluate the "toxins" you feel after having dealt with toxic people.

They can be anyone, worse yet, they can be people you have to deal with every day: your supervisors, teachers, coworkers, and, regrettably, even your family and friends. People with all the warmth and congeniality of—an electric eel! People you cannot escape, but could certainly do with less of. You may eventually have to explain to them, "You make me sick—literally—you make me feel anxious, and tense. You make my stomach ache, my head hurt, and my nose twitch"…whatever! Selye's studies of the human stress response state that we are emotional beings and that our interpersonal relations are guided more by our emotions than by our logic.[8] Having to cope with difficult people and personalities is one of the "greatest causes of distress."[9] The formula seems complete; people who cause you stress, leave you with distress—the bad kind you really want to avoid.

WHO ARE "THE JONESES" ANYWAY?

Perhaps you think you have never met "The Joneses," but I bet we have all met them at some point in our lives.

You're pulling the weeds from your front garden, when you see your neighbors pull up in their new SUV. It's big, shiny, air-conditioned, and has all the electronic gadgets you could dream of. You wave, smiling a nod of approval, then go to the garage to find your pruning shears—that is when it hits you. You cannot help noticing your aging car. It needs new snow tires this year, and there's an odd noise in the front end—could be the axel, or brakes, (oh, not the brakes again!). Then, you take another glance across the yard at the gleaming new SUV. You are caught! You know you want one, too. Your mind does the math, trying to figure it into your budget. "What budget?" you ask—there isn't one! Certainly not for a new vehicle, but look at those rims…and you can bet the air conditioning is ice cold. So, you do a little financial tango with the bank, some refinancing of this and that and a few weeks later, you're beaming with pride as you drive past your neighbor—in your new SUV. Sucker!

Your teenaged son comes home from school and announces that his best friend's parents just got one of those new plasma TVs and a state of the art DVD player with surround sound—they have transformed their living room into a theatre. He then begins to mutter under his breath about the lousy TV and VCR (VCR?…get with the times!) in the living room. For a nanosecond, you consider an upgrade, but decide there is nothing wrong with the TV and VCR (albeit prehistoric) that you have. No one is missing any important programs on the setup you have. Your son decides he will be watching a lot more of "the game" over at his friend's house from now on. Penny-pincher!

"Hurry in!"

"Buy now!"
"Save on two!"
"Beat the rush!"
"Avoid disappointment—come early!"
"Prices have never been lower!"
"The sale ends Saturday!"

Every time advertisers try to lure us in to buy something, there is a time limit attached to it, as though a stampede of shoppers will beat us to it if we don't go NOW! Advertise a great sale, and the masses will converge as though Moses were leading them to freedom (let my people go…and shop!). If we don't have it, we have to get it, and if we don't need it, we will find some reason to need it. The disease of "stuff" and "never enough" has infected just about everyone. We might, however, call it materialism.

There is nothing really wrong with wanting more or acquiring things to make us happy. The retiree who has worked years to afford a luxury sailboat deserves it. The family who decides to entertain the kids at home with a swimming pool—why not? The graduate who has spent seven years, during college and university, riding a bicycle deserves a new car with that first successful job! Why not? Why not, if you can afford it? But many cannot afford it, so they put it on credit, mortgage it, charge it, consolidate, refinance—whatever they can do to get it. Many people are living outside their means. Too many! And it is causing serious debt and even more serious *STRESS*.

Money was the second largest stressor in the group of women I had researched. There seems to be an ever-present expectation to keep up with "The Joneses," but what about the cost? Competition is stressful to begin with, but when you are competing to obtain the biggest and the best, it can cause more stress than it is worth. We are born with nothing, and we cannot bring everything to the grave. He who dies with the most toys—still dies! Whoever made that up was dead-on! What good is it to have everything, yet become so stressed in pursuing it that you do not live long enough to enjoy it? Things can make us happy, but if acquiring things makes us sick, then, what good is that?

Money cannot buy happiness, and it cannot buy your health. Sure, it might offer you the finest treatment, the best doctors, even a posh suite at a top notch clinic, but if the stress of "getting" makes you sick, it is just not worth it.

A friend once described a young man she knew who was all about "what" he had. He had a big, beautiful home, a manicured yard, a luxury car, a celebrity wardrobe, and a classy SUV for his wife to showcase their kids around in. He had it all, it seemed, but really, it all had him! His workday often stretched past sunset, while his wife spent many hours alone at home. He had bought his house with a second mortgage (probably at loan-shark interest rates). His vacations extended no farther than the end of his driveway. He was a prisoner of his own things. He was living above his means, and if that is living, I say, "Thanks, but no thanks."

THE PRESSURE

I had barely said, "I do" when the questions started. The first thing practically everyone asked me just after I got married, besides when the babies were coming, was "Have you bought a house yet?" To which I replied, "No, we're in no rush." Then I'd have to stand there and listen to their poetic reasoning about it being in our best financial interest to buy; otherwise, we were just "throwing our money away" on rent. I knew the story, but we were not ready to purchase a home. While interest rates were lower, the housing market had never been higher. Besides, too many times I witnessed the perils of "too much, too soon." I knew many people who had married, bought a house, a dog, a new car, a big-screen TV, had their first child, and were working on their second all in their first year of marriage!

In all truth, these women described that they felt saddled with debt and overwhelmed with responsibilities. They had not vacationed in a long time and hardly ever had quality time with their spouses. Now, it was all pills and bills, diapers and dishes! So when people were pressuring me and asking why I had not followed suit, I would reply that we were taking our time and that we did not want to jump into debt right away. I am glad my husband and I did not run into debt like so many young people whose marriages suffer because of it. We have had time to acquire quality things for our home and to enjoy ourselves and get to know each other as a married couple. We have had time to travel together and pursue our individual interests. When I lived on my own, as a teenager and into my twenties, my apartment consisted of little more than a bed, an old black-and-white TV, and a lawn chair! I was even paying a student loan for a college diploma I never received! I knew what it was like to live way below the norm, and in debt, but I was also cautious not to start living way above our means. Measuring up to others' standards and keeping up with everyone else is just too much stress.

Present: Tense!

Poverty, healthcare, politics, taxes, economics, education, preservatives, pollution, and germs are just a few of our daily stressors. As a society, we struggle with new sources of stress and anxiety that previous generations did not have to face. Moreover, it all makes for a more tense society. I believe women in particular feel the extremes because of the multiple roles they play and responsibilities they hold. Within the last few years, we have had to face new stressors, which remind us we cannot be too safe or prudent anymore. In the last decade, new fears have gripped Western society including West Nile Virus, sudden acute respiratory syndrome (SARS), mad-cow disease, terrorism, and blackouts. It seems we are programmed for fear and anxiety more than ever before.

The first thought many people had just moments after the power outage on August 14, 2003 was that this was another terrorist attack. You could cut the tension in the air with a knife! It was the largest blackout in North American history with some fifty million people without power. It extended all along the North Eastern United States and Canada, including Ontario and Quebec. I admit, terrorism flashed in my mind, too. However, once this threat had been ruled out, many actually began to enjoy this mini electrical holiday, gathering for impromptu BBQ's, chatting with neighbors by candlelight, and rediscovering heavenly constellations suddenly visible in the uncommon darkness.

Nonetheless, the first reaction was fear. We have become a society on edge, poised for the next disaster; waiting for the sky to fall—hyper-vigilant people—worried, anxious, and ready to run! As fear infects our minds, it also affects us metabolically and physiologically. Studies show that fear directly relates to the initiation of the stress hormone response, preparing us for whatever behavioral response may be necessary.[10] Fears contribute to the stress that wears us down each day. Fear and continued pressures to accomplish more and be more combine to create chronic stress that is often unrelenting. I am not talking of the hairpin turns of sudden acute stress, like your child breaking an arm, your husband bringing his new boss home for dinner, or your mother-in-law angry at the door, but rather the long, winding road of chronic stress.

We need more time to accomplish things, so we need more medication to keep us going so that we can be better mothers, wives, or employees so that if things get tense and the world starts to crumble, we can try to save everyone. And, if there's time, we'll even try to save ourselves. These are unrealistic demands—overwhelming needs! Women frequently feel the need to please everyone, even at their own expense. At least, this was my case. Not only was I looking after my own needs, I also felt I needed to please everyone else. I was convinced that if I did not make it, did not amount to something, then people would see me as a failure. Despite all my hard work and accomplishments, performance anxiety lingered. I was not only discouraged about my past, but I was worried about my future as well. The expectations I had were making me sick.

Superwoman was not real—she was a comic strip character. What makes a woman super is not what she does, but who she is. I was trying to be the comic strip character, and it is what I see other women doing all the time. They suffer the same plight as mine: to be more, to do more, to have more, and to look great while we're at it! If we do not accomplish it all, we worry about it all. Yet, where is worry going to get us? There is much wisdom in the biblical teachings of Jesus to his disciples when he says:

> Do not worry about your life, what you will eat or drink or wear; is life not more important than food and the body more important than clothes? Who of you by worrying can add a single hour to your life? Therefore, do not worry about tomorrow, for tomorrow will worry about itself. Each day has enough trouble of its own.[11]

We're Overworked

One day an article on CNN.com caught my attention. It suggested that America should consider adapting to the European way of life, by working less and living more, using France as an example. The article did not suggest that we become slack, but rather that we balance our lives better. Western society has often debated the idea that the European lifestyle promotes greater, longer-lasting health. It was interesting to note that France participates in eleven public holidays per year, and that their national law allows for a minimum of five weeks paid vacation with a thirty-five-hour work week.[12] This is a remarkable difference from Canada and the United States. The North American workweek is much longer, and typical vacation periods in Canada are ten days or two weeks. Americans enjoy even fewer at only eight days on average.[13]

In my life, the equilibrium between work and life has been severely imbalanced, and I was feeling its effects. Balance is much easier said than done. Try telling a single mother with two young children and a full-time job to enjoy more time for herself, and she will likely laugh in your face. Try to explain a balanced life to a family with two working parents, children, and bills to pay. On an interesting episode of America's popular relationship expert, Dr. Phil, he stated that research found that a woman who raises three children experiences the equivalent of two full-time jobs! That is just raising the kids—never mind her other part-time or full-time jobs outside the home. Let's do the math. That means a sixteen to eighteen hour day of work! Where is a woman supposed to find time to get in the thirty minutes of daily cardio exercise or two to three sessions of strength training per week that many health professionals would advise?

I agree with this advice; however, if a woman wants to keep fit, stay healthy, maintain her weight, and reduce stress, twenty-four hours in a day just won't do! Then, of course, there are the healthy meals to prepare because fast food and processed foods are not good for you. Who has that kind of time? Work is not just the eight hours you spend at your job; it is whatever time it takes to prepare for the day, including travel to and from your job. It seems there is less and less time for family and oneself. Again, time was the most requested commodity of my research group—especially "alone" time. It was also the main cause of guilt for these women. Never mind buying shoes, shopping sprees, or a movie with friends—what made these women feel the most guilt was simply spending time away from other responsibilities to enjoy solitude or personal time. They did not feel guilty about what they were enjoying or buying for themselves. Instead, the women described feeling as though they needed to hurry back.

One woman described feeling so overwhelmed with her responsibilities and work that she felt she had "lost her identity and could not remember the last time she did something for herself." This made me feel genuinely sorry for her and all the women who share her plight. I am sure other women feel this way, too. Women face a time famine and this is reflected their health. With shocking statistics on obesity, heart disease, cancers depression and "obscure" illnesses like chronic fatigue, fibromyalgia, and syndrome x (metabolic syndrome), it is clear that a significant imbalance exists between work and life for women.

Let us consider again Maslow's theory and Hans Selye's studies, which argue that if you overwork something, it simply breaks down. For a moment, imagine a utopia in which women could be both successful in their careers and readily available for their families. OK,—on another planet, maybe, but let's just pretend for a moment. Imagine a workday that would allow mothers (particularly of younger, school-aged children) to be home to see their children off to school each morning, as well as be there when they return in the afternoon. The school day begins around 8:30 AM and ends anywhere from 3:00–3:30 PM for most North American children. Why then, does a workday often begin earlier and end much later? Given that many parents are not home until five, six or seven o'clock at night, it is no wonder North American cultures have increasing problems with children's issues like obesity, drugs, alcohol, mental and emotional dysfunction, young offenders, bullying, and teenaged suicide. But, that is a whole other book in itself.

Imagine how families would benefit from having a parent at home to greet their child from school. Imagine how a women's self esteem would improve if she was able to balance work and family commitments, without being stretched as impossibly thin as most women are in our current system. This new balance would also alleviate the self-destructive guilt that many women feel by choosing to work while trying to be a good parent. Imagine the moaning employers not wanting to hire these women. In any case, society has to get its head out of the proverbial sand and cooperate more with working women, especially if they want to combat the worsening social problems, the alarming health problems, and the collapsing families of our overworked and over-stimulated society.

It is one thing to agonize over these problems. It is another thing to work together to develop ways to fix these problems, yet until we address the real issues and roots of women's stress and sickness, we are just pedaling backwards. We need to create a family-friendly workplace and offer more part-time opportunities, flexible hours, and job-sharing options for women with young families. Too many employers are stuck on a full-time, nine-to-five, Monday-to-Friday workweek. There are fewer options for part-time employment without suffering consequences like the loss of seniority and benefits. If employers, politicians, and people in general considered the adverse impact of stress on our health care, social benefits, and crumbling family dynamics, I am convinced society would be better as a whole.

The statistics do not lie and women's health issues are climbing to epidemic proportions. The diseases killing women are not just in the drinking water! I believe chronic stress contributes to these illnesses more than we would like to think. As scientifically advanced as we are, we still lack the balance we need in order to live healthy lives.

Women are still the principal caregivers for children in the home. Additionally, women want to feel capable of having a career and contributing financially to their households. In modern society, you would think we would have worked out something more agreeable by this point. A woman's career might span some forty-plus years, while child rearing and family responsibilities might take less than half of that time before the nest is empty. These children, by the way, are our future—our leaders and decision makers—the ones who will have to govern and lead our society. Hopefully, they will also be able to care for us when we are older.

It's a woman's right to have a family. She should not have to decide between a career and children. She should not have to leave her infant alone all day in a daycare facility, pay exorbitant amounts for babysitters, or forfeit her job. Our society needs change. We need to provide more options for balance. Maybe at first, employers and politicians might think greater benefits and options are not feasible, or are even impossible, but many people scoffed at the idea of walking on the moon and snickered at the thought of discovering DNA. Impossible became possible because we made it work and believed that what we were doing was best for humankind. Do we regret these decisions?

I know many young, married women, who are afraid to start a family because they feel it would be overwhelming to juggle both family and career. Perhaps this is one reason why women are waiting longer to get married and the birthrate is getting lower. In Canada, the birthrate has declined significantly; as of 2001, it stood at 1.51 children per woman.[14] By the time a woman finishes university, finds a job, gets married and thinks of starting a family, she is into her late twenties or early thirties. Many women often struggle with wanting children, yet they need the income from their jobs, too. They worry about who will watch their kids while they are at work or about how they could not afford to work because their wages would be spent on childcare. If a woman decides to stay at home, she feels the threat of losing pace with the workforce, falling behind in skills and technology, and having difficulty re-entering the job market afterward. Author M. Sara Rosenthal sums it up clearly in her book *Women Managing Stress*, "today, the mother who does not work is considered a statistical anomaly."[15] Yet, she goes on to explain that married, employed women feel torn between their responsibilities at work and at home and that this is largely contributing to their stress.[16]

(*BODY*) IMAGE IS EVERYTHING!

"Honey, do I look fat?" Most men wince when the woman in their life asks this question; however, it may be that more men are asking women this question nowadays. Today, body image is everything! You cannot turn on the television or browse through a bookstore without being flooded with images of "perfection" and "beauty." There are more products and procedures for maintaining youth and appearance available now than ever before. Gone are the days of simply applying a moisturizer and flossing before bedtime. Enter the age of Botox injections, laser teeth whitening, micro-dermabrasion skin resurfacing, laser eye surgery, and implants for just about every body part! There is a whole world of makeover magic tantalizing women (and men) to embrace the fountain of youth, and for those who can afford it, it is working like magic! It doesn't stop with adults either as more youths and teens are jumping on the makeover bandwagon when their finances allow for it.

Although self-image and body image are two very different things (thanks Dr. Phil!), they are also closely related. They go hand-in-hand. For example, imagine two women having lunch together. One is a grocery clerk and the other is a CEO of a successful company. The first woman is overweight, rather unattractive and dressed in an outdated outfit; whereas, the second woman is slender, attractive, and dressed in cashmere. Who do you suspect is the CEO? Ask anyone this question and they will probably say the second woman in cashmere is the CEO and the unattractive woman is the grocery clerk.

Value judgments and success are often measured by what we look like. If we look good, then we must be good. There is much more pressure for women to look attractive than there is for men, although men, too, can suffer from low self-esteem due to appearance. Our society focuses too much more attention on women's appearances than on their physical and emotional health. Star-studded, red carpet waifs may appear to be healthy, but we need to place more emphasis on optimum health and proper weight. Trying to obtain the look of magazine images—stick-thin models and airbrushed beauties—is unrealistic. Many women fall into a depression for this reason. After having children and working so much, they often resemble more of Babar than of Bardot!

When their body image suffers, they do not feel pretty, young, or sexy anymore. When they do not believe they look good anymore, they feel negative about their self-image as well. Being overweight suddenly makes them feel stupid, ugly, and unmotivated, even though most women are probably overworked and chronically stressed. Women pay a heavier price than men do when it comes to body image and self-esteem. When men are overweight, people often dismiss it as the product of too much "R & R" (a few too many good times with the boys). In addition, their size can be misinterpreted as muscular and strong.

Many men can be overweight and know it, yet they seem to be better at separating their body image from their self-image. "I might be a little chunky, but I'm a darn good golfer." They can still maintain a stronger self-image while admitting they need to shed a few pounds. And with more testosterone than women, shedding those few pounds is often much easier for the guys. They do not place the emphasis on their appearance as much as women. With this, men do not feel the sting of competition amongst their male peers about their looks as much as women do. Men seem to compete more in areas of strength, sport, endurance, and material acquisition, while women notoriously compete more by comparing their appearances.

Men can get away with carrying a few extra pounds. But a bigger woman? "What a cow" is one insult that comes to mind. We attach much harsher stereotypes to overweight women. Obese women are seemingly less accepted. In a society obsessed with appearance, it is little wonder that young girls, even under the age of ten, have become more concerned about their appearance. You see them sporting thong underwear peaking above skin-tight jeans or wearing teeny-tiny, ill-fitting clothes attempting to mimic their idols. The number of cases of eating disorders and illnesses including anorexia and bulimia are rising—even developing popularity through clubs and Internet sites. Dieting is common among elementary and teen-aged girls. Research has indicated that eating disorders are reaching "epidemic" proportions and that children are succumbing to the pressures of body image even before reaching high school.[17] Sex sells and being sexy is where it's at. Never mind being healthy, we need to be sexy—pencil thin with no fat and all the latest fashion styles. Unfortunately, women, or should I say, girls, are starting younger and younger, drawn into the fashion frenzy and hype of being thin and beautiful, at virtually any cost—even to their own health.

8

Simplify

Men, for the sake of getting a living, forget to live.

—Margaret Fuller

Simplifying your life sounds—well, simple; however, it can take a lot of effort and attention. When you consider the effort and expense, it sounds like more stress than it is worth; however, in the words of Thomas Edison, "opportunity is missed by most people because it is dressed in overalls and looks like work."[1] If only we would treat simplifying our lives as an opportunity to educate ourselves about health and well being. I know I had to work hard at simplifying my life, but I do not regret one second I spent working at it.

Being busy has become second nature, and all too often, it's hard to say no. Yet, attitudes are changing. Some people are adopting a new attitude deciding to slow down, enjoy life, and particularly focus on family life. People have created organizations to re-establish quality family time. "Putting Family First," an organization growing in the United States and programs like "Family Night" created in Ridgewood, New Jersey, are on the forefront of new family values. These organizations and programs are devoted to reclaiming family time, opening communication lines between family members, and actually sitting down to have meals together. Studies in North America have confirmed that over the past two decades, the incidence of families eating dinner together has actually decreased by 33 percent. Over-scheduling of activities and the frantic pace of everyday life has diminished both the quality and quantity of family time. Parents are starting to realize that it is much harder to pass down family values and traditions to their children when there is no downtime.[2]

Rest and relaxation, in our society, has become something pretty much limited to our vacation time. Having said that, the most common thing I hear people say, and I'm often guilty of this, too, is that they have planned so much during their vacation that they actually look forward to returning to work to get a rest! Somewhat ironic, don't you think?

9

The Wisdom of Self-Education and Prevention

Wisdom preserves the life of its possessor.

—Ecclesiastes, 7:12

With more demand for newer and advanced technology, we have become a society that needs to reinvent itself in order to face new challenges each day. Just think about the rapid changes in computers and software development, communications technology, and even automobiles. The things we use and rely on for daily living are always changing, demanding that we keep pace as well. The same is true with our health, only, we seem to spend more time and money on maintaining things like our cars with oil changes, tune ups and repairs, than we do with our bodies; it is sad, but true.

Just as a car cannot go forever without maintenance, neither can we. We practice prevention better with our cars than we do with our health. Each autumn I take my car in for a new undercoating to protect it from the effects of the sand, salt, ice and snow of Canadian winters. I give my car oil changes routinely and check regularly to make sure the air conditioning, electrical system, and engine are all running properly. It is a very healthy car! On the other hand, many of us are not accustomed to taking care of ourselves until we are sick or feeling symptoms of illness. If we took the same approach to our health as we do with our belongings, we might agree that "an ounce of prevention is worth a pound of cure." We suffer from our lack of knowledge, and, all too often, it is with our health.

Lack of knowledge leaves you like a sitting duck, and women are particularly vulnerable to this. Need a scenario? I will admit, I used to be a victim of "car repair ignorance," but years of repairs later, I am no longer a pushover. Ladies, have you ever taken your car to a repair shop or garage and tried to describe the problems you are having? The mechanic nods, appearing sympathetic; however, when you are describing the "thud" sound in the "thinga-ma-jiggy" and the fluid leaking from "that round black thing," the mechanic knows you have no idea what's wrong or how to fix it. Then you leave your car in their capable hands, only to return to pick up your "fixed" car and a repair bill that makes you wonder if you should have sold a kidney or left behind your first born child!

Naïve? Gullible? Well, I would rather call it uneducated. If you have no idea what is wrong or how to fix something, all too often, you fall prey to those who do, and sometimes they take advantage of your ignorance or do not take you seriously. Am I suggesting the medical world does this? Not really. I will just say that when it comes to health and ambiguous symptoms, the doctors' responses are often it is just a phase, a woman thing," or "all in your head." In his book, *The Stress of Life*, Dr. Hans Selye states: "In order to adjust or repair a machine, we first have to know how it works. This is of course also true of the stress machinery with which man combats the wear and tear of whatever he does in this world"[1] Doctors often give the quick-fix solutions because it's the fastest and easiest thing to do, but that just masks the underlying problem, especially with the complex symptoms that chronic stress can produce.

On the other hand, a woman who enters a garage with at least an educated guess about her car troubles, for instance, "I think it is the radiator—it is overheated and green stuff is coming out at the front," will not be such a target for profit. The mechanic knows she has a clue as to the problem, so it is harder for him to take advantage of her. I use this scenario because car repairs are one of the biggest complaints I hear from women who have been "had." This is not to suggest that all auto shops take advantage of uninformed women, but it does frequently happen.

The same principal is true of health and stress. Once you have an understanding about the nature of chronic stress, you can begin to identify the areas of your life that it could be restricting, even damaging. With knowledge of the actual stress process in your body, you can develop strategies to relieve stress and maintain a balanced life. If we accept stress with the attitude that everyone has it and there is nothing we can do about it, then we must suffer the consequences.

Stress is a multifaceted and complex phenomenon that operates differently in each person. We do not need to feel intimidated, vulnerable, or "in the dark" about chronic stress. Knowing how your body works is the first step to being healthy. How can we fix something if we do not know how it works? Self-education about health not only supports your experiences with knowledge, but also supports your understanding of your symptoms and gives you the opportunity to discuss it more openly with your health-care professional. Knowledge also opens up doors to exploring alternative health care practices and medicines that could give you the relief you are really looking for.

An Ounce of Prevention...

Have you ever seen anyone water a tree by spraying the leaves and branches? Western society often practices medicine this way. They water the leaves and branches. This might work in theory, by allowing the water to drip down to the roots, but it is much more effective to water the roots at ground level. We are accustomed to treating disease only after it has manifested itself in the body. We spend more than half of our health care costs on treating symptoms to keep people alive and only a small portion on prevention.[2] Yet, in other areas, we practice prevention all the time. We install anti-virus software to protect against computer viruses and keep a spare tire in the trunk in case of a flat. We take an umbrella to work just in case it rains. We brush our teeth to prevent cavities.

However, when it comes to our overall health, we usually wait until illness has a face before we accept it is time to take better care of ourselves. I felt I was too young to have so many symptoms. Deciding to change my lifestyle became essential to better health; after all, I was not getting any younger. I also made the effort to prevent further damage. I changed my diet and exercised more often. I have risen to the challenge of becoming a regular runner. I am no marathon runner yet, but you never know. More importantly, I learned to accept who I was despite my troublesome past. I learned to relax and to make time to do the things I have always enjoyed. I did this because it was essential to my health, not because I had nothing else to do. If you think that taking time for the things you enjoy is frivolous or insist that you do not have the time, then you will never do it.

There is that time thing again! You can always find something else to do. You have to make the time. Whether I mop the floors today or tomorrow is not important, my linoleum will survive if it is not scrubbed right away! Each day, I make it a priority to relax and do something I enjoy, even if only for a short while. I have made exercise as important as anything else. Finding the time was not my trouble, it was convincing myself to put other things aside and just do it! When I was younger and in school, I would take on extra work hours. Now, however, exercise is as important to me as working, eating, or brushing my teeth—it is just something else I need to do each day.

Regular exercise has been my defense against chronic stress because it is a great way to release tension and frustration. It also gave me a sense of accomplishment, something I had not felt in a long time. I started to think more positively about myself. It helped me realize what chronic stress was doing to me. I resolved that it was not about my past or what mistakes I had made; it was now about the rest of my life. I was determined to live as content and healthy as I possibly could. Prevention was now more crucial to my life than ever before.

A New Attitude!

It is never too late to be what you might have been.

—George Elliot

With a new attitude, I decided it was time to change more than just my daily routine, exercise regiment, and diet. It was time to cast off my thoughts of failure. In my heart, I knew I was not a failure. It was time to claim what was rightfully mine. I began by getting the recognition and fair academic evaluation that I deserved. I had to muster up the courage to drive up the long, winding driveway of the college I had attended more than a decade earlier. But this time, I was filled with self-confidence and determination—not humiliation. I talked to the department coordinator and explained my dilemma from many years ago. She was understanding and explained that there were several other complaints regarding the instructor who had failed me. She carefully studied my transcript and agreed that my other marks did not reflect a failed student; however, I was still missing the half-credit necessary to obtain my diploma.

A few years earlier at the university where I worked, I had taken a computer course for my own general interest. I finished the course with an "A," and because I was formally registered as a student, I earned a half-credit for this course. I proposed that the coordinator transfer this half-credit from the university to fulfill the necessary credit on my college transcript. With the approval of the college, I could obtain my diploma. The college accepted this and within a few days, I was granted my college diploma! I felt vindicated and had finally graduated! The stress of this injustice had weighed so heavily on me for years. Now, I felt I got what I deserved. This was one stressor I will never regret letting go.

NATURAL APPROACH TO A NATURAL PHENOMENON

One of the first duties of the physician is to educate the masses not to take medicine.

—Sir William Osler

Stress is natural. We are supposed to experience stress. Although we are equipped to deal with it, we are not meant to live with it continuously. With my numerous diagnoses, depression may have seemed the most reasonable explanation, but I was really living a lifestyle of chronic stress. When this pushed me to the end of my wits, I decided to explore natural medicine and alternative practices. I was very skeptical and close-minded to many aspects of natural medicine, but as I began to understand the nature of the treatments and methods that naturopathic doctors use, I began to let down my guard.

Natural Medicine

The leaves of the trees are for the healing of the nations...
—Revelation 22:2

Natural medicine, or alternative medicine, is not new. It has been around for thousands of years. Beginning with Hippocrates around 400 BC, it gained more popularity throughout each century up to the eighteen hundreds. During this time, a German doctor named Benedict Lust introduced naturopathic practices to the United States, coining the name naturopathy. Beginning in 1902, students in America could graduate as practitioners of natural medicine. By the nineteen twenties, natural medicine practices found their way into Canada.[3] Since the nineteen sixties, researchers and practitioners have seen major research and advancements in natural medicine.[4]

Naturopathy is gaining popularity in Western culture; however, many people have mixed reactions to it and are still questioning its validity for treating illness and disease. I was one of those skeptics—until I witnessed the results of natural medicine in my own life. Once I mentioned to my supervisor that I had a very open mind about alternative medicine and naturopathic doctors, to which he replied, "Oh that...that stuff, hmm...I don't know about that." I assured him it was effective for me. My husband was a little suspicious of naturopathy, too. One day after returning from an appointment with my naturopath, he asked, "How was your visit with the psychopath?" Amused, I replied, "She's not a psychopath, she's a naturopath." He responded, "Whatever, you know what I mean."

To many people, holistic and alternative medicine is, well, weird. Instead, most of us have become accustomed to "allopathic" or conventional medicine. Naturopathy is based on six principles: (1) do no harm—respect the body and use non-invasive treatments; (2) harness the healing power of nature—believe the body has the inherent ability to heal itself; (3) treat the whole person—mind, body, and spirit; (4) prevent illness—encourage prevention as the best medicine; (5) identify and treat the cause of the disease—don't suppress symptoms, rather treat the root cause; and (6) view doctors as teachers—help patients understand the cause of their illness and encourage self-education and responsibility.[5]

Homeopathy, a special kind of natural medicine, is based on the idea that "like cures like" or the "Law of Similars" developed by Samuel Hahnemann over two hundred years ago. In other words, homeopaths give minute doses of substances, derived from plants, animals, and minerals, to sick people to invoke the body's own healing process that would otherwise *cause* those specific symptoms in a healthy person. Homeopathy is still highly controversial. The philosophy of homeopathy is based on the premise that the absence of illness does not indicate health, but that true health is three-fold: physical, mental, and emotional. It is based on restoring health not just treating symptoms.[6] Symptoms may be the prime indicators of illness, but most often, symptoms manifest only after the disease has begun its course.

Alternative practices include everything from aromatherapy to biofeedback, yoga, massage, art, music therapy, water therapy, Reiki, meditation, cleansing, acupuncture, and the list goes on. More and more patients are turning to alternative medicines and therapies. Europeans and Eastern cultures have practiced alternative health care for years, and it is now beginning to surge in North America. Patients not able to find relief using conventional methods have been exploring alternative medicine. Many find that a combination of both conventional and alternative medicine works best.

Alternative and natural methods are no guarantee for relieving the symptoms of chronic stress. It takes time, as with any illness, but it also requires more action and responsibility by the patient. Unlike pharmaceuticals and conventional medicine, natural medicine "requires time for self-education."[7] I took the time—many months, in fact—to understand what was going on with my health. I was not sick in any clinical sense, but I was convinced I had some sub-clinical illness draining me of my youth, energy, sleep, and vitality. I could have been well on my way to developing many of the illnesses that are plaguing women today.

Most importantly, once I decided to take action, I was able to realize that I was not crazy. My symptoms were real, not psychosomatic. I was not imagining anything; it was not "all in my head." This knowledge alone spelled relief for me. I also took comfort in finally having real medical doctors confirm that I was not suffering from depression. Afterwards, I wondered why it had taken so long to figure out what was wrong with me. I believe, in part, it was because I felt intimidated because was not a doctor or medical professional. At first, I was diving into medical information I could barely understand, but the more I searched, the more I could understand. I did not need a PhD to figure it out. I am not suggesting that you become your own doctor—by all means, no! On the other hand, I am encouraging you to learn about your body and health. Regardless of your background and formal education, you can work with your doctors to better understand yourself and your health. Ultimately, you are the judge of your health. With today's availability of information, you can learn in ways that even non-professionals can relate. I have surprised myself with how much I have come to understand.

Now, like the woman with a few clues about her car trouble, I enter my doctor's office these days with a decent knowledge of my health. I am no longer insecure because of ignorance or intimidated by my doctor's expertise. If I do not understand something, I look it up and continue to research it until I find an explanation that is simple enough for me to understand. Then I am better informed before I talk with my doctor. I know now that many of my health problems arose because I assumed that being young meant being healthy, but chronic stress is harmful at any age.

To briefly recap the course of chronic stress in my life: a high-stress lifestyle plagued me for a long time. I was experiencing many symptoms I could not connect to a particular problem. I had difficulty sleeping, likely due to high cortisol levels, which contributed to chronic fatigue. High cortisol levels also prompted sugar and carbohydrate cravings, causing weight gain. Due to poor sleep and lack of relaxation, I was also experiencing headaches and muscle stiffness. My immune system was suppressed by stress and high cortisol, which lowered my ability to fight off pathogens—like *Candida*. Thus, the vicious cycle continued, producing many symptoms difficult to diagnose. Depression seemed the only explanation. Yet, I refused to accept this diagnosis and am thankful for it. I am thankful I took the road less traveled, educating myself about the problems associated with chronic stress. It has made all the difference.

TOTAL HEALTH

A valuable lesson I've learned is that being healthy means more than not being sick. True health combines the many aspects of our being—our body, mind, emotion, and spirit. They are intricately linked. Dysfunction in one area can readily spread, afflicting other areas. Though the benefits of exercise, healthy eating, and adequate rest are crucial, balancing our emotions and calming our spirit are essential to our health as well. Too often, we equate true health only with our outward appearance.

However, there is a whole world of unseen, subtle processes happening which can manifest disease. My childhood experiences did not equate disease, but they set the stage for the path of chronic stress. Learning to parent myself and having lost a child were huge emotional struggles, and they deteriorated my physical health as well. My attitude of failure from my college experience was more of a mental struggle; however, it too, ravaged my health. Eventually, it seems the body pays the highest price.

TRY SAILING!

Change is good. We have heard that before, but we do not often embrace this attitude with our health. Taking care of yourself is…well, another thing to do in our hectic day. Very few of us need more to do; however, subtle changes can make huge differences. I have learned to incorporate changes slowly into my life and am feeling the benefits many fold. I did not go radical—move to the hills, stop shaving my legs, and milk my own herd of goats. I just made simple, small changes that yielded good results. Making small, gradual changes can improve your health and reduce stress in such a beneficial way that you will barely notice making any change at all. The key is to set your eyes on your goal and try to stay focused.

Reflecting upon writing this book, I am reminded of my sailing instructor. A few years ago, I decided to take sailing lessons in an attempt to try something different. I always wanted to sail. Though I did not end up yachtswoman of the year, I did earn my "White Sail" level three certificate. From this course, I learned a valuable lesson that I apply to almost everything. When the winds and waves would lead my little boat astray, I became nervous about capsizing or flipping the boat.

Frantically, my small crew and I would begin fumbling around to keep the thing afloat.

The interesting thing about sailing is that to get where you want to go, you cannot just assume the path of least resistance. The obstacles in your way, wind, waves, and other boaters, become the very things that determine your course and direction. If you are going across the lake, you have to tack and jibe, literally zigzagging your way, using the winds to help you get there. You cannot just beeline straight across—you cannot sail that way. All too often, the instructor would call out, "Keep your eye on your goal," the goal being the place where we had decided to sail to that day. We would pick a point on the other side of the lake. Mine was always a brightly colored flag on some lovely cottage dock way on the other side. This became our focal point, our goal. Reaching our destination required a series of steps: little twists and turns, here and there, dodging obstacles in our way, but above all, we had to keep an eye on our goal. If we lost sight of our focal point, well, then we were thankful our instructor had a towrope on his boat.

The sailing analogy is kind of like life, especially when assuming responsibility for your health. It requires taking those little steps, making small changes, a few turns here, a couple of twists there—the whole time, trying to keep control and to focus on improving. Eventually, you learn to ride the waves, go with the winds, and get to the other side—you learn how to take better care of yourself, and you begin to feel better. You have to reprogram your mind and habits, but the health benefits are many fold. Almost 80 percent of medical appointments are stress-related. Combine that figure with soaring health care costs, doctor shortages, and fear of privatization to see that health is becoming more of a personal responsibility. However, you should not take responsibility for something you do not know anything about.

In a society driven by convenience, availability, and instant gratification, we have neglected to inform ourselves about the major health risks women face. Likewise, most women do not really know what chronic stress (distress) is and how seriously it can affect their health. Many women seem to just accept their doctors' diagnosis whatever it is and end up developing long-term dependencies on drugs.

There is nothing wrong with pharmaceuticals; they can be very useful and effective when we use them properly; however, it is clear we are almost unconsciously addicted to quick-fix treatments—we don't focus on the root of the problems. With the potential damage that chronic stress can cause, it should be clear that we need to learn more about stress and bring these issues to the forefront.

We need new attitudes toward health and new health initiatives. Women, in particular, need to speak out to their doctors asking them to provide more options and a better understanding of health and treatments. Besides, medical professionals have evaluated women's health in the shadows of men's health for too long. Clearly, women are uniquely different from men. Although men and women suffer similar illnesses, a woman's body is designed differently from a man's, and chronic stress and resulting hormonal changes affect women differently than men. Essentially, we need to redefine women's health so that we can better serve their needs. Women have made remarkable progress in establishing themselves in society; however, we need to focus more attention on why women are so sick, chronically stressed, and, literally, starved for time.

10

Conclusion

After all my research and reading and after taking back control of my life and health, I can honestly say, I have never felt better! I have more energy and vitality than I can ever remember having. The tension headaches? Hardly ever, and I know what brings them on and how to control them. The insomnia? Do not ask me at 3:18 AM, I am probably asleep! If I do wake up, I have learned not to panic and that I can usually get back to sleep. The prescriptions? I only take them when absolutely required. Most importantly, I am no failure and never was! I spent so many nights crying, pleading and begging God and the doctors to help me, to cure me, to find some kind of relief. I wanted some cosmic healing to fall from the heavens—a miracle. The miracle I received was far better than I could have imagined. In my pursuit of better health, I acquired the one thing necessary to find the causes of what had tormented me for so long. I had learned how to learn.

Knowledge was the essential ingredient to my health. This was the key to my cure. It was my healing and my deliverance. Even my begging God to understand what was wrong became clear: He wanted me to understand my health, my body, and me and to learn how to change in order to be healthy. Begging for a magic-wand cure would have neither allowed me to understand how I got this way, nor compelled me to take control and to change my lifestyle to feel better. It would have been another quick fix—a divine quick fix maybe, but a quick fix just the same. For years, I thought God did not want to bother with me, but now I realize, not only did God care about me, but also he wanted me to care about myself. I had asked him to tell me, show me, and teach me what was wrong, and I believe he did. Educating myself about my own health, led by his grace and guidance is how I got better.

I now firmly believe that prevention is the key and that a combination of natural and conventional medicines produces the best results. The tinnitus—it is gone, and candida—it is a sneaky one, but I now know how to detect it, to control it, and to avoid what could exacerbate it.

The most encouraging thing of all is that my latest test results revealed that my cortisol levels have returned to normal—to the immense surprise of my doctor and his nurse! They both asked quite ecstatically, "What did you do to lower your cortisol like that?" I told them about all my research, my new understanding of health, and my efforts to change my diet, lifestyle, and attitude. I described the natural therapies and medicines that I took, as well as how I educated myself about vitamins, minerals, and supplements that would help me. I am thirty-five now, and I have my whole life ahead of me! Am I cured? Well, yes—I would say I am. The path toward good health is open to you, too.

As for my past, that is where I have chosen to leave it—in the past. The experiences of a fearful and unstable childhood set chronic stress in motion, which deteriorated my health. Yet, forgiveness is a wonderful thing. It should be spelled F-R-E-E-D-O-M because that is exactly what it offers. Grudges, anger, and resentment are exhausting and corrosive. Like an anchor, they weigh you down and will eventually degrade your health. I was not going to let the way I had grown up ruin the life ahead of me. With the help of therapy aimed at restoring my emotions, I have formed an amicable relationship with my parents.

Even since I began researching for this book, the stress hormone cortisol has steadily made headlines with regard to health issues. Many products and therapies specifically designed to reduce the effects of high levels of cortisol are now available. I would encourage anyone experiencing chronic stress and its subsequent negative health effects to research these products and discuss potential therapies with their doctors and health care providers. Stress will always be a part of our lives, but we do not have to live with the health consequences that follow it.

Did you notice the image on the cover of this book? She is the "Miss" of mysterious symptoms. She was me and could be you or anyone who bears the mark of mystery illness. She is the iconic woman enduring misdiagnosis after misdiagnosis of chronic stress symptoms with no real understanding of her condition.

Not often would someone crowned with a title be willing to give it up, especially if they earned it with hard work and determination; however, the title I was wearing I earned through years of chronic stress. Today, I have traded my symptoms for wisdom, and the new title I bear is one of knowledge of my health. I do not intend to give up this new title.

As for the old title, it is with great pride, satisfaction, and outright joy that I relinquish my crown, as I am no longer *MISS DIAGNOSED*.

REFERENCES

Introduction:

1. Posen, D., *The Little Book of Stress Relief* (Key Porter Books, 2003), 21.

2. *Taber's Cyclopedic Medical Dictionary* (Philadelphia: F.A. Davis, 1989).

3. *The Random House Dictionary*, 9th ed. (New York: Ballentine Books, 1988).

4. Vanderhaeghe, L., "Stress: At the Root of Women's Health Issues," *Healthy Immunity*, no. 8 (2003): 1.

Chapter 4:

1. *The Random House Dictionary*, 9th ed. (New York: Ballentine Books, 1988).

2. http://www.ncptsd.org/facts/general/fs_what_is_ptsd.html

3. Selye, H., *Stress without Distress,* (New York: Harper & Row, 1974), 20.

4. Sathicq, L., "Putting on Weight: Blame It on Your Hormones," *Good Medicine* (July 2003): 34.

5. Sapse, A. T., "Cortisol, High Cortisol Diseases and Anti-cortisol Therapy," *Psychoneuroendocrinology* 22, no. 1 (1997): S3–S10.

6. Maleskey, G., M. Kittel and others, *The Hormone Connection: Revolutionary Discoveries Linking Hormones and Women's Health Problems* (Rodale, 2001), 273.

7. McEwen, B. and E. Norton-Lasley, *The End of Stress As We Know It* (Washington DC: Joseph Henry Press, 2002), 24.

8. Ibid., 25.

9. Selye, H., *The Stress of Life,* (New York: McGraw-Hill, 1974), 56.

10. Ibid., 73.

11. Stress Management, http://stress.about.com/library/weekly/aa012901a.htm.

12. Sapolsky, R. M., *Why Zebra's Don't Get Ulcers: An Updated Guide to Stress, Stress-Related Diseases, and Coping,* (W.H. Freeman and Co., 1998), 245.

13. Heart and Stroke Foundation of Canada, "Report Cards on Health—Stress Threatening Canadian's Health, Heart and Stroke Foundation Warns," February 2, 2000, http://www.heartandstroke.ca

14. Hancock, M., "Young and Stressed," *Alive* 251 (September 2003): 49.

15. McEwen, B. S., "Protective and Damaging Effects of Stress Mediators," Seminars in Medicine of the Beth Israel Deaconess Medical Centre, *New England Journal of Medicine* (Jan. 15, 1998): 171.

16. Ibid., 172.

17. McEwen, B. S. and E. Norton Lasley, *The End of Stress As We Know It* (Washington DC: Joseph Henry Press, 2002), 4.

Chapter 5:

1. Simpson, James B., *Simpson's Contemporary Quotations* (Houghton Mifflin, 1988).

2. Selye, H., *The Stress of Life* (New York: McGraw-Hill, 1974), 55.

3. The McGraw-Hill Companies.

4. Selye, H., *Stress without Distress* (New York: Harper & Row, 1974), 17–19.

5. Ibid., 19.

6. Ibid., 13.

7. www.hope.edu.academic/psychology/335/webrep2/stress2.html

8. Selye, H., *Stress without Distress* (New York: Harper & Row, 1974), 12.

9. *The Random House Dictionary,* 9th ed. (New York: Ballentine Books, 1988).

10. Maté, G., *When the Body Says No: The Cost of Hidden Stress* (Toronto: Alfred A. Knopf, 2003), 32.

11. Selye, H., *Stress without Distress* (New York: Harper & Row, 1974), 15.

12. Rosenthal, M. S., *Women Managing Stress: A Sourcebook of Natural Solutions* (Prentice-Hall, 2002), 4–5.

13. Lesch Kelly, A., "Sick of Stress: Improve Your Outlook Along with Your Health," *Woman's Day,* (May 6, 2003): 48.

14. Rosenthal, M. S., *Women Managing Stress: A Sourcebook of Natural Solutions,* (Prentice-Hall, 2002), 4.

15. http://www.factmonster.com/ce6/sci/A0824782.html

16. Maleskey, G., M. Kittel and others, *The Hormone Connection: Revolutionary Discoveries Linking Hormones and Women's Health Problems,* (Rodale, 2001), 273.

17. *Time Magazine,* "Women and Heart Disease," http://www.time/com/covers/1101030428/story.html

18. Naugle, W. and D. Chen, "It's Time to Save Your Life," *Glamour,* (October 2003): 208.

19. Chrousos, G. and P. Gold, "The Concept of Stress and Stress System Disorders," *JAMA,* 267, no. 9 (Mar. 4, 1992): 1244.

20. Maté, G., *When the Body Says No, The Costs of Hidden Stress,* (Toronto: Alfred A. Knopf, 2003), 28.

21. Talbott, Shawn M., *The Cortisol Connection: Why Stress Makes You Fat and Ruins Your Health—and What You Can Do about It,* 1st ed., (California: Hunter House, 2002), 15.

22. DeMarco, C., "Avoiding Adrenal Exhaustion," *Alive,* no. 245 (March 2003): 59.

23. Talbott, Shawn M., *The Cortisol Connection: Why Stress Makes You Fat and Ruins Your Health—and What You Can Do about It,* 1st ed., (California: Hunter House, 2002), 9.

24. Talbott, Shawn M., private communication.

25. Talbott, Shawn M., *The Cortisol Connection: Why Stress Makes You Fat and Ruins Your Health—and What You Can Do About It,* 1st ed., (California: Hunter House, 2002), 29.

26. Ibid., 23.

27. Elkind, D., *The Ties That Stress: The New Family Imbalance,* (Harvard Press, 1995), 182.

28. Dobson, J., "Focus on the Family," Bulletin, September 2002.

29. McEwan, B. S., "Protective and Damaging Effects of Stress Mediators," *Seminars in Medicine of the Beth Israel Deaconess Medical Center* 338 (Jan. 15, 1998): 176.

30. Ibid., 171.

31. Colbert, D., *What Would Jesus Eat? The Ultimate Program for Eating Well, Feeling Great and Living Longer* (Nashville: Thomas Nelson, 2002), 189.

32. Hemels, M, G. Koren and T. Einarson, "Increased Use of Antidepressants in Canada: 1981–2000," *Annals of Pharmacotherapy* 36, no. 9 (2002): 1375–1379.

33. Peskett, T., "Common Prescriptions Linked to Cancer—Are You at Risk?" *Alive* 246 (April 2003): 53.

34. DeGrandpre, R., *Ritalin Nation: Rapid-Fire Culture and the Transformation of Human Consciousness* (New York: Norton, 2000), 174.

35. Earle, R., Canadian Institute of Stress, private communication.

36. Waterhouse, D., *Outsmarting Female Fatigue: 8 Energizing Strategies for Lifelong Vitality*, (New York: Hyperion Books, 2001), 188–189.

37. Ibid., 188.

38. Vanderhaeghe, L., *Alive* 252 (October 2003): 56.

39. Ibid., 55.

40. Epel, E., R. Lapidus, B. McEwen and K. Brownell, "Stress May Add Bite to Appetite in Women: A Laboratory Study of Stress-Induced Cortisol and Eating Behavior," *Psychoneuroendocrinology* 26 (2001): 37–49.

41. Bjorntorp, P., "Do Stress Reactions Cause Abdominal Obesity and Co-morbidities?" *Obesity Rev.* 2 (2001): 80.

42. Bjorntorp, P., "Body Fat Distribution, Insulin Resistance and Metabolic Disease," *Nutrition* (1997): 795.

43. Ibid., 797.

44. Kalyan, S., "The Syndrome Marked X," *Alive* 246 (April 2003): 56.

45. Bjorntorp, P., "Body Fat Distribution, Insulin Resistance and Metabolic Disease," *Nutrition* (1997): 800–801.

46. Bjorntorp, P., "Do Stress Reactions Cause Abdominal Obesity and Co-morbidities?" *Obesity Rev.* 2 (2001): 73.

47. Bauman, A. and others, *Fight Fat: Secrets to Successful Weight Loss* (Rodale Press, 1998), 149.

48. Epel, F., et al., "Stress and Body Shape: Stress-Induced Cortisol Secretion Is Consistently Greater among Women with Central Fat," *Psychosomatic Med.* 62 (2000): 623.

49. Colbert, D., *What Would Jesus Eat? The Ultimate Program for Eating Well, Feeling Great and Living Longer* (Nashville: Thomas Nelson, 2002), xi.

50. Ibid.

51. Colbert, D., *What Would Jesus Eat? The Ultimate Program for Eating Well, Feeling Great and Living Longer* (Nashville: Thomas Nelson, 2002), 5.

52. Wickelgren, I., "Obesity: How Big a Problem?" *Science* 280 (May 29, 1998): 1364.

53. The World Health Organization's World Health Report 2002, http://temagami.carleton.ca/jmc/cnews/15112002/connections.shtml

54. Statistics Canada, Canadian Community Health Survey, 2003, http://www.statcan.ca/Daily/English/040615/d040615b.htm

55. Maté, G., *When the Body Says No: The Cost of Hidden Stress* (Toronto: Alfred A. Knopf, 2003), 95.

56. *Stress Management,* "Cortisol: The "Stress Hormone" Part II: Abnormal Cortisol Levels," http://www.stress.about.com/library/weekly/aa012901b.htm

57. Al-Damluji, S., T. Iveson, J. Thomas, D. Pendlebury, L. Rees, and G. Besser, "Food-Induced Cortisol Secretion Is Mediated by Cen-

tral Alpha-1 Adrenoceptor Modulation Pituitary ACTH Secretion," *Clin. Endocrinology* 26 (1987): 629–636.

58. Talbott, Shawn M., *The Cortisol Connection: Why Stress Makes You Fat and Ruins Your Health—and What You Can Do about It,* 1st ed. (California: Hunter House, 2002), 15.

59. Svec, F. and A-L Shawar, "The Acute Effect of a Noontime Meal on the Serum Levels of Cortisol and DHEA in Lean and Obese Women," *Psychoneuroendocrinology* 22, no. 1 (1997): S117.

60. Graci, S., "Insurance Plan for a Lifetime," *Alive,* no. 246 (April 2003): 87.

61. Rabin, B., *Stress, Immune Function and Health: The Connection* (Wiley, 1999), 19.

62. Rouse, J., Overtraining and Life's Olympics, Be Alive & Well, Your Health and Wellness Guide, 1st ed., (2003), 4.

63. Rabin, B., *Stress, Immune Function and Health: The Connection* (Wiley, 1999), 20.

64. Vellucci, S. V., "The Autonomic and Behavioural Responses to Stress," in *Stress, Stress Hormones and the Immune System,* ed. J. C. Buckingham, G. E. Gillies and A. Cowell (Wiley, 1997), 50.

65. Cowell, A., J. C. Buckingham and G. E. Gillies, "In Vivo and In Vitro Methods for Assessing Neuroendocrine Function," in *Stress, Stress Hormones and the Immune System,* ed. J. C. Buckingham, G. E. Gillies and A. Cowell, (Wiley, 1997), 129.

66. Buckingham, J. C., A. Cowell and G. E. Gillies, "The Neuroendocrine System: Anatomy Physiology and Responses to Stress," in

Stress, Stress Hormones, and the Immune System, ed. J. C. Buckingham, G. E. Gillies and A. Cowell, (Wiley, 1997), 10.

67. Goulding, N. J. and R. J. Flower, "Glucocorticoids and the Immune System," in *Stress, Stress Hormones and the Immune System,* ed. J. C. Buckingham, G. E. Gillies and A. Cowell, (Wiley, 1997), 221.

68. Aspinall, R. J., "The Immune System," in *Stress, Stress Hormones and the Immune System,* ed. J. C. Buckingham, G. E. Gillies and A. Cowell, (Wiley, 1997), 91.

Chapter 6:

1. Trowbridge, J. P. and M. Walker, *The Yeast Syndrome* (New York: Bantam Books, 1986), 30.

2. Ibid., 12.

3. Crook, W. G., *Tired—So Tired and the "Yeast Connection,"* (Jackson, Tennessee: Professional Books, 2001), 42.

4. Igram, C., *The Cure Is in the Cupboard* (Illinois: Knowledge House, 1997), 49.

5. Trowbridge, J. P. and M. Walker, *The Yeast Syndrome* (New York: Bantam Books, 1986), 15.

6. Ibid., xvi.

7. Ibid.

8. Crook, W. G., *Tired—So Tired and the "Yeast Connection,"* (Jackson, Tennessee: Professional Books, 2001), 155.

9. Watson, B, "Candida: Controlling the Yeast", *Alive* 273, (July, 2005): 42.

10. Igram, C., *The Cure Is in the Cupboard* (Illinois: Knowledge House, 1997), 19.

11. Ibid., 17.

12. Trowbridge, J. P. and M. Walker, *The Yeast Syndrome* (New York: Bantam Books, 1986), 10.

13. Igram, C., *The Cure Is in the Cupboard* (Illinois: Knowledge House, 1997), 20.

14. Ibid., 21.

15. Ibid.

16. Trowbridge, J. P. and M. Walker, *The Yeast Syndrome* (New York: Bantam Books, 1986), 61.

17. Ibid., 18.

18. Crook, W. G., *Tired—So Tired and the "Yeast Connection,"* (Jackson, Tennessee: Professional Books, 2001), 157.

19. Ibid., 159.

20. Dr. Michael Biamonte, private communication.

21. Rubin, J., "The Yeast/Fungus Link: The True Cause of Candida and Fungal Infections," *Alive* 247 (May 2003): 50–54.

22. Crook, W. G., *Tired—So Tired and the "Yeast Connection,"* (Jackson, Tennessee: Professional Books, 2001), 156.

23. Rubin, J., "The Yeast/Fungus Link: The True Cause of Candida and Fungal Infections," *Alive* 247 (May 2003): 54.

24. Cater, R. E., "Chronic Intestinal Candidiasis as a Possible Etiological Factor in the Chronic Fatigue Syndrome," *Med. Hypothesis* 44 (1995): 513.

Chapter 7:

1. DeGrandpre, R., *Ritalin Nation—Rapid Fire Culture and the Transformation of Human Consciousness* (New York: W.W. Norton, 2000), 16.

2. Ibid., 81.

3. Ibid., 104.

4. http://www.web.utk.edu/~gwynne/maslow.HTM

5. http://www.stoptellingustobe.com/axletree/

6. Sheehan, D. V., *The Anxiety Disease and How to Overcome It* (Scribner, 1984), 12.

7. Peele, S., *Diseasing of America—Addiction Treatment out of Control,* (Massachusetts: Lexington, DC Heath & Co., 1989), 14.

8. Selye, H., *Stress without Distress* (New York: Harper & Row, 1974), 61.

9. Ibid.

10. Shulkin, J., "Allostasis: A Neural Behavioral Response," *Hormones and Behavior* 43, no. 1 (January 2003): 21–27.

11. Matthew 6:25–34, NIV.

12. Anderson, G. T., "Should America be France?" http://www.money.cnn.com/2003/10/06/pf/work_less/index.html

13. Ibid.

14. Statistics Canada.

15. Rosenthal, M. S., *Women Managing Stress: A Sourcebook of Natural Solutions* (Prentice-Hall, 2002), 112.

16. Ibid., 106.

17. Black, S., "Starving in Silence: Eating Disorders Take a Heavy Toll on Students Academically as Well as Physically." http://www.asbj.com/2002/03/0302research.html

Chapter 8:

1. McWilliams, J. and P. McWilliams, *Do It! Let's Get Off Our Butts: A Guide to Living Your Dreams* (Prelude Press, 1991), 420.

2. Cassidy, A., "Family Comes First," *Women's Faith & Spirit*, Premier ed. (2003): 58–61.

Chapter 9:

1. Selye, H., *The Stress of Life* (New York: McGraw-Hill, 1974), 402.

2. Cook, M., "The Root of Great Health," *Health 'N Vitality*, no. 16 (February 2003): 24.

3. Conn, H., "Best of Both Worlds: Bridging the Medical Divide," *Alive* 247 (May 2003): 36.

4. http://www.healthunlimitedministries.org/naturopathic_health.html

5. Craig, C., "Naturopathy Fundamentals," *Alive* (April 2003): 30.

6. Conn, H., "Best of Both Worlds: Bridging the Medical Divide," *Alive* 247 (May 2003): 36.

APPENDIX

Suggested Readings

Colbert, D., *What Would Jesus Eat? The Ultimate Program for Eating Well, Feeling Great and Living Longer,* Nashville: Thomas Nelson, 2002.

DeGrandpre, R., *Ritalin Nation: Rapid-Fire Culture and the Transformation of Human Consciousness,* New York: Norton, 2000.

Elkind, D., *The Ties That Stress: The New Family Imbalance,* Harvard Press, September 1995.

Igram, C., *The Cure Is in the Cupboard,* Illinois: Knowledge House, 1997.

Maleskey, G., M. Kittel and others, *The Hormone Connection: Revolutionary Discoveries Linking Hormones and Women's Health Problems,* Rodale: Prevention Health Books for Women, 2001.

Maté, G., *When the Body Says No: The Cost of Hidden Stress,* Toronto: Alfred A. Knopf, 2003.

McEwen, B. and E. Norton-Lasley, *The End of Stress as We Know It,* Washington DC: Joseph Henry Press, 2002.

Peele, S., *Diseasing of America—Addiction Treatment Out of Control,* Massachusetts: Lexington, DC Heath & Co., 1989.

Posen, D., *The Little Book of Stress Relief,* Key Porter Books, 2003.

Rosenthal, M. S., *Women Managing Stress: A Sourcebook of Natural Solutions,* Canada: Prentice-Hall, 2002.

Sapolsky, R. M., *Why Zebra's Don't Get Ulcers: An Updated Guide to Stress, Stress-Related Diseases, and Coping,* W.H. Freeman and Co., 1998.

Selye, H., *Stress without Distress,* New York: Harper & Row, 1974.

Sheehan, D. V., *The Anxiety Disease and How to Overcome It,* Scribner, 1984.

Talbott, S. M., *The Cortisol Connection: Why Stress Makes You Fat and Ruins Your Health—and What You Can Do about It,* 1st ed., California: Hunter House, 2002.

Trowbridge, J. P. and M. Walker, *The Yeast Syndrome,* New York: Bantam Books, 1987.

Waterhouse, D., *Outsmarting Female Fatigue: 8 Energizing Strategies for Lifelong Vitality,* New York: Hyperion Books, New York, 2001.

978-0-595-35688-1
0-595-35688-5

he United States
0009B/40/A